I0015129

Machine Learning for Healthcare Analytics Projects

Build smart AI applications using neural network
methodologies across the healthcare vertical market

Eduonix Learning Solutions

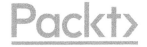

BIRMINGHAM - MUMBAI

Machine Learning for Healthcare Analytics Projects

Copyright © 2018 Packt Publishing

All rights reserved. No part of this book may be reproduced, stored in a retrieval system, or transmitted in any form or by any means, without the prior written permission of the publisher, except in the case of brief quotations embedded in critical articles or reviews.

Every effort has been made in the preparation of this book to ensure the accuracy of the information presented. However, the information contained in this book is sold without warranty, either express or implied. Neither the author(s), nor Packt Publishing or its dealers and distributors, will be held liable for any damages caused or alleged to have been caused directly or indirectly by this book.

Packt Publishing has endeavored to provide trademark information about all of the companies and products mentioned in this book by the appropriate use of capitals. However, Packt Publishing cannot guarantee the accuracy of this information.

Commissioning Editor: Sunith Shetty
Acquisition Editor: Shweta Pant
Content Development Editor: Nathanya Dias
Technical Editor: Utkarsha Kadam
Copy Editor: Safis Editing
Project Coordinator: Kirti Pisat
Proofreader: Safis Editing
Indexer: Priyanka Dhadke
Graphics: Jisha Chirayil
Production Coordinator: Nilesh Mohite

First published: October 2018

Production reference: 2091118

Published by Packt Publishing Ltd.
Livery Place
35 Livery Street
Birmingham
B3 2PB, UK.

ISBN 978-1-78953-659-1

www.packtpub.com

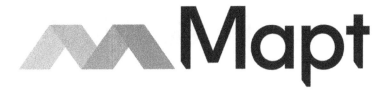

`mapt.io`

Mapt is an online digital library that gives you full access to over 5,000 books and videos, as well as industry leading tools to help you plan your personal development and advance your career. For more information, please visit our website.

Why subscribe?

- Spend less time learning and more time coding with practical eBooks and Videos from over 4,000 industry professionals

- Improve your learning with Skill Plans built especially for you

- Get a free eBook or video every month

- Mapt is fully searchable

- Copy and paste, print, and bookmark content

Packt.com

Did you know that Packt offers eBook versions of every book published, with PDF and ePub files available? You can upgrade to the eBook version at `www.packt.com` and as a print book customer, you are entitled to a discount on the eBook copy. Get in touch with us at `customercare@packtpub.com` for more details.

At `www.packt.com`, you can also read a collection of free technical articles, sign up for a range of free newsletters, and receive exclusive discounts and offers on Packt books and eBooks.

Contributor

About the author

Eduonix Learning Solutions creates and distributes high-quality technology training content. Our team of industry professionals have been developing workforces for more than a decade. We aim to teach technology the way it is used in industry and the professional world. We have a professional team of trainers for technologies ranging from mobility, web enterprises, and database and server administration.

Packt is searching for authors like you

If you're interested in becoming an author for Packt, please visit `authors.packtpub.com` and apply today. We have worked with thousands of developers and tech professionals, just like you, to help them share their insight with the global tech community. You can make a general application, apply for a specific hot topic that we are recruiting an author for, or submit your own idea.

Table of Contents

Preface

Machine learning in the healthcare domain is booming because of its ability to provide accurate and stable techniques. Machine learning algorithms provide strategies to deal with a variety of structured, unstructured, and semi-structured data. This book is packed with new approaches and methodologies to create powerful solutions for healthcare analytics.

This book will implement key machine learning algorithms and their use cases using a range of libraries from the Python ecosystem. We will build five end-to-end projects within the organization to evaluate the efficiency of artificial intelligence applications when carrying out simple and complex healthcare analytics tasks. Each project will help you to delve deep into newer and better ways to manage insights and handle healthcare data efficiently. We will use machine learning to detect cancer in a set of patients using the SVM and KNN models. Apart from that, we will create a deep neural network in Keras to predict the onset of diabetes on a huge dataset of patients. We will also learn how to predict heart diseases using neural networks.

By the end of this book, you will learn how to address long-standing challenges, provide specialized solutions to deal with them, and carry out a range of cognitive tasks in the healthcare domain.

Who this book is for

If you are a data scientist, machine learning engineer, or a healthcare professional who wants to implement machine learning algorithms to build smart AI applications, then this is a book for you.

Basic knowledge of Python or any programming language is expected to get the most from this book.

What this book covers

Chapter 1, *Breast Cancer Detection*, will show you how to import data from the UCI repository. In this chapter, we will name the columns (or features) and put them into a pandas DataFrame. We will learn how to preprocess our data and remove the ID column. We will also explore the data so that we know more about it. We will also see how to create histograms (so that we can understand the distributions of the different features) and a scatterplot matrix (so that we can look for linear relationships between the variables). We will learn how to implement some testing parameters, build a KNN classifier and an SVC, and compare their results using a classification report. Finally, we will build our own cell and explore what it would take to actually get a malignant or benign classification.

Chapter 2, *Diabetes Onset Detection*, covers the building of a deep neural network in Keras. We will explore the optimal hyperparameters using the scikit-learn grid search. We will also learn how to optimize a network by tuning the hyperparameters. In this chapter, we will explore how to apply the network to predict the onset of diabetes in a huge dataset of patients.

Chapter 3, *DNA Classification*, will show how to predict the functional outcome—or a promoter/non-promoter —for a DNA sequence from E. coli bacteria with 96% accuracy. We will look at how to import data from a repository and how to convert textual inputs to numerical data. We will then learn to build and train classification algorithms and compare and contrast them using the classification report.

Chapter 4, *Diagnosing Coronary Artery Disease*, will show how to use sklearn and Keras, how to import data from a UCI repository using the pandas read_csv function, and how to preprocess that data. We will then learn how to describe the data and print out histograms so we know what we're working with, followed by executing a train/test split with the model_selection function from sklearn.

Furthermore, we will also learn how to convert one-hot encoded vectors for a categorical classification, defining simple neural networks using Keras. We will look at activation functions, such as softmax, for categorical classifications with categorical_crossentropy. We will also look at training the data and how we fit our model to our training data for both categorical and binary problems. Ultimately, we will look at how to do a classification report and an accuracy score for our results.

Chapter 5, *Autism Screening with Machine Learning*, will show how to predict autism in patients with approximately 90% accuracy. We will also learn how to deal with categorical data; a lot of health applications are going to have categorical data and one way to address them is by using one-hot encoded vectors. Furthermore, we will learn how to reduce overfitting using dropout regularization.

To get the most out of this book

This book will help you to build real-world machine learning solutions across the healthcare vertical using NumPy, pandas, matplotlib, scikit-learn, and so on. You need not have any prior knowledge before exploring this book. You will get well versed on how exactly machine learning is implemented to evaluate the efficiency of AI apps, and how to carry out simple-to-complex healthcare analytics tasks. This is a perfect entry point packed with practical examples to carry out a range of cognitive tasks. By the end of this book, you will have learned how to address long-standing challenges in the healthcare domain, and produce solutions for dealing with them.

Download the example code files

You can download the example code files for this book from your account at www.packt.com. If you purchased this book elsewhere, you can visit www.packt.com/support and register to have the files emailed directly to you.

You can download the code files by following these steps:

1. Log in or register at www.packt.com.
2. Select the **SUPPORT** tab.
3. Click on **Code Downloads and Errata**.
4. Enter the name of the book in the **Search** box and follow the onscreen instructions.

Once the file is downloaded, please make sure that you unzip or extract the folder using the latest version of:

- WinRAR/7-Zip for Windows
- Zipeg/iZip/UnRarX for Mac
- 7-Zip/PeaZip for Linux

The code bundle for the book is also hosted on GitHub at `https://github.com/ PacktPublishing/Machine-Learning-for-Healthcare-Analytics-Projects`. In case there's an update to the code, it will be updated on the existing GitHub repository. We also have other code bundles from our rich catalog of books and videos available at `https://github. com/PacktPublishing/`. Check them out!

Download the color images

We also provide a PDF file that has color images of the screenshots/diagrams used in this book. You can download it here: `https://www.packtpub.com/sites/default/files/ downloads/9781789536591_ColorImages.pdf`.

Conventions used

There are a number of text conventions used throughout this book.

`CodeInText`: Indicates code words in text, database table names, folder names, filenames, file extensions, pathnames, dummy URLs, user input, and Twitter handles. Here is an example: "We will then rename that file `autism_detection`."

A block of code is set as follows:

```
import sys
import pandas as pd
import sklearn
import keras
print 'Python: {}'.format(sys.version)
print 'Pandas: {}'.format(pd.__version__)
print 'Sklearn: {}'.format(sklearn.__version__)
print 'Keras: {}'.format(keras.__version__)
```

When we wish to draw your attention to a particular part of a code block, the relevant lines or items are set in bold:

```
[default]
exten => s,1,Dial(Zap/1|30)
exten => s,2,Voicemail(u100)
exten => s,102,Voicemail(b100)
exten => i,1,Voicemail(s0)
```

Any command-line input or output is written as follows:

```
jupyter lab
```

Bold: Indicates a new term, an important word, or words that you see onscreen. For example, words in menus or dialog boxes appear in the text like this. Here is an example: "If we go into **Files**, we will see all the files that we have in the directory, as shown in the following screenshot."

 Warnings or important notes appear like this.

 Tips and tricks appear like this.

Get in touch

Feedback from our readers is always welcome.

General feedback: If you have questions about any aspect of this book, mention the book title in the subject of your message and email us at customercare@packtpub.com.

Errata: Although we have taken every care to ensure the accuracy of our content, mistakes do happen. If you have found a mistake in this book, we would be grateful if you would report this to us. Please visit www.packt.com/submit-errata, selecting your book, clicking on the Errata Submission Form link, and entering the details.

Piracy: If you come across any illegal copies of our works in any form on the Internet, we would be grateful if you would provide us with the location address or website name. Please contact us at copyright@packt.com with a link to the material.

If you are interested in becoming an author: If there is a topic that you have expertise in and you are interested in either writing or contributing to a book, please visit authors.packtpub.com.

Reviews

Please leave a review. Once you have read and used this book, why not leave a review on the site that you purchased it from? Potential readers can then see and use your unbiased opinion to make purchase decisions, we at Packt can understand what you think about our products, and our authors can see your feedback on their book. Thank you!

For more information about Packt, please visit packt.com.

1
Breast Cancer Detection

Machine learning, a subset of **artificial intelligence (AI)**, has taken the world by storm. Within the healthcare domain, it is possible to see how machine learning can make manual processes easier, providing benefits for patients, providers, and pharmaceutical companies alike. Google, for example, has developed a machine learning algorithm that can identify cancerous tumors on mammograms. Similarly, Stanford University has developed a deep learning algorithm to identify skin cancer.

In this chapter, we will discuss how one can use machine learning to detect breast cancer. We will look at the following topics:

- Objective of this project
- Detecting breast cancer with SVM and KNN
- Data visualization with machine learning
- Relationships between variables
- Understanding machine learning algorithms
- Training models
- Predictions in machine learning

Objective of this project

The main objective of this chapter is to see how machine learning helps detect cancer through the SVM and KNN models. The following screenshot is an example of the final output that we are trying to achieve in this project:

```
In [6]:   # Let explore the dataset and do a few visualizations
          print(df.loc[10])

          # Print the shape of the dataset
          print(df.shape)

          clump_thickness             1
          uniform_cell_size           1
          uniform_cell_shape          1
          marginal_adhesion           1
          single_epithelial_size      1
          bare_nuclei                 1
          bland_chromatin             3
          normal_nucleoli             1
          mitoses                     1
          class                       2
          Name: 10, dtype: object
          (699, 10)
```

We will receive the information shown in the preceding screenshot for approximately 700 cells in our dataset. This will include factors such as clump_thickness, marginal_adhesion, bare_nuclei, bland_chromatin, and mitoses, all of which are properties that would be valuable for a pathologist. In the screenshot, you can see that the class is 4, which means that it is malignant; so, this particular cell is cancerous. A class of 2, on the other hand, would be benign, or healthy.

Now, let's take a look at the models that we will be training as the chapter progresses in the following screenshot:

```
In [10]:  # Define models to train
          models = []
          models.append(('KNN', KNeighborsClassifier(n_neighbors = 5)))
          models.append(('SVM', SVC()))

          # evaluate each model in turn
          results = []
          names = []

          for name, model in models:
              kfold = model_selection.KFold(n_splits=10, random_state = seed)
              cv_results = model_selection.cross_val_score(model, X_train, y_train, cv=kfold
              results.append(cv_results)
              names.append(name)
              msg = "%s: %f (%f)" % (name, cv_results.mean(), cv_results.std())
              print(msg)

          KNN: 0.962468 (0.018609)
          SVM: 0.958929 (0.029934)
```

Based on the cell's information, both models have predicted that the cell is cancerous, or malignant. In this project, we will go through the steps required to achieve this goal. We will start by downloading and installing packages with Anaconda, we will move on to starting a Jupyter Notebook, and then you will learn how to program these machine learning models in Python.

Detecting breast cancer with SVM and KNN models

In this section, we will take a look at how to detect breast cancer with a **support vector machine** (**SVM**). We're also going to throw in a **k-nearest neighbors** (**KNN**) clustering algorithm, and compare the results. We will be using the conda distribution, which is a great way to download and install Python since conda is a package manager, meaning that it makes downloading and installing the necessary packages easy and straightforward. With conda, we're also going to install the Jupyter Notebook, which we will use to program in Python. This will make sharing code and collaborating across different platforms much easier.

Now, let's go through the steps required to use Anaconda, as follows:

1. Start by downloading `conda`, and make sure that is in your `Path` variables.
2. Open up a Command Prompt, which is the best way to use `conda`, and go into the `Tutorial` folder.
3. If `conda` is in your `Path` variables, you can simply type `conda install`, followed by whichever package you need. We're going to be using `numpy`, so we will type that, as you can see in the following screenshot:

```
Anaconda Prompt

(base) C:\Users\test>D:

(base) D:\>cd D:\Tutorial

(base) D:\Tutorial>conda install numpy
```

If you get an error saying that the command `conda` was not found, it means that `conda` isn't in the `Path` variables. Edit the environment variables and add `conda`.

4. To start the Jupyter Notebook, simply type `jupyter notebook` and press *Enter*. If `conda` is in the path, Jupyter will be found, as well, because it's located in the same folder. It will start to load up, as shown in the following screenshot:

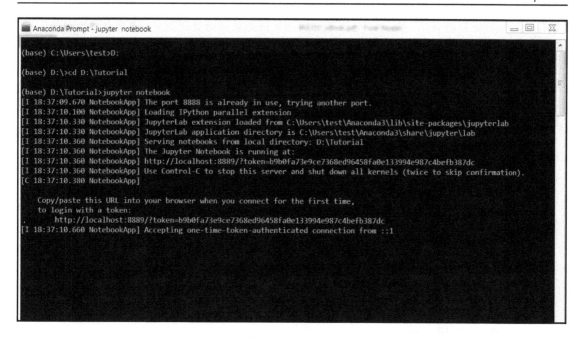

The folder that we're in when we type `jupyter notebook` is where it will open up on the web browser.

5. After that, click on **New,** and select **Python [default]**. Using **Python 2.7** would be preferable, as it seems to be more of a standard in the industry.
6. To check that we all have the same versions, we will conduct an import step.
7. Rename the notebook to `Breast Cancer Detection with Machine Learning`.
8. Import `sys`, so that we can check whether we're using Python 2.7.

 We will need to import `numpy` for computational operations and arrays, `matplotlib` for plotting, `pandas` to handle the datasets, and `sklearn`, to get the machine learning packages.

9. We will import `numpy`, `matplotlib`, `pandas`, and the `sklearn` packages and print their versions. We can view the changes in the following screenshot:

```
In [1]:  import sys
         import scipy
         import numpy
         import matplotlib
         import pandas
         import sklearn

         print('Python: {}'.format(sys.version))
         print('scipy: {}'.format(scipy.__version__))
         print('numpy: {}'.format(numpy.__version__))
         print('matplotlib: {}'.format(matplotlib.__version__))
         print('pandas: {}'.format(pandas.__version__))
         print('sklearn: {}'.format(sklearn.__version__))

         Python: 3.6.6 |Anaconda, Inc.| (default, Jun 28 2018, 11:27:44) [MSC v.1900 64
         bit (AMD64)]
         scipy: 1.1.0
         numpy: 1.15.0
         matplotlib: 2.2.2
         pandas: 0.23.3
         sklearn: 0.19.1
```

To run the cell in Jupyter Notebook, simply press *Shift + Enter*. A number will pop up when it completes, and it'll print out the statements. Once again, if we encounter errors in this step and we are unable to import any of the preceding packages, we have to exit the Jupyter Notebook, type `conda install`, and mention whichever package we are missing in the Terminal. These will then be installed. The necessary packages and versions are shown as follows:

- Python 2.7
- 1.14 for NumPy
- Matplotlib
- Pandas
- Sklearn

The following screenshot illustrates how to import these libraries in the specific way that we're going to use them in this project:

```
In [2]:  import numpy as np
         from sklearn import preprocessing, cross_validation
         from sklearn.neighbors import KNeighborsClassifier
         from sklearn.svm import SVC
         from sklearn import model_selection
         from sklearn.metrics import classification_report, accuracy_score
         from pandas.plotting import scatter_matrix
         import matplotlib.pyplot as plt
         import pandas as pd

             C:\Users\test\Anaconda3\lib\site-packages\sklearn\cross_validation.py:41: Depr
             ecationWarning: This module was deprecated in version 0.18 in favor of the mod
             el_selection module into which all the refactored classes and functions are mo
             ved. Also note that the interface of the new CV iterators are different from t
             hat of this module. This module will be removed in 0.20.
               "This module will be removed in 0.20.", DeprecationWarning)
```

In the following steps, we will look at how to import the different arguments in these libraries:

1. First, we will import NumPy, using the command `import numpy as np`.
2. Next, we will import the various classes and functions in `sklearn` - namely, `preprocessing` and `cross_validation`.
3. From neighbors, we will import `KNeighborsClassifier`, which will be KNN.
4. From `sklearn.svm`, we will import the **support vector classifier** (**SVC**).
5. We're going to do `model_selection`, so that we can use both KNN and SVC in one step.
6. We will then get some metrics, in which we will import the `classification_report`, as well as the `accuracy_score`.
7. From `pandas`, we need to import plotting, which is the `scatter_matrix`. This will be useful when we're exploring some data visualizations, before diving into the actual machine learning.
8. Finally, from `matplotlib.pyplot`, we will import `pandas as pd`.
9. Now, press *Shift + Enter*, and make sure that all of the arguments import.

 You may get a deprecation warning, as shown in the preceding screenshot. That is because some of these packages are getting old.

10. Now that we have all of our packages set up, we can move on to loading the dataset. This is where we're going to be getting our information from. We're going to be using the UCI repository, since they have a large collection of datasets for machine learning, and they're free and available for everybody to use.

11. The URL that we're going to use can be imported directly, if we type the whole URL. This is going to import our dataset with 11 different columns. We can see the URL and the various columns in the following screenshot:

```
In [3]:  # Load Dataset
         url = "https://archive.ics.uci.edu/ml/machine-learning-databases/breast-cancer-wisconsin/breast-cancer-wisconsin.data"
         names = ['id', 'clump_thickness', 'uniform_cell_size', 'uniform_cell_shape',
                 'marginal_adhesion', 'single_epithelial_size', 'bare_nuclei',
                 'bland_chromatin', 'normal_nucleoli', 'mitoses', 'class']
         df = pd.read_csv(url, names=names)
```

We will then import the cell data. This will include the following aspects:

- The first column will simply be the ID of the cell
- In the second column, we will have clump_thickness
- In the third column, we will have uniform_cell_size
- In the fourth column, we will have uniform_cell_shape
- In the fifth column, we will have marginal_adhesion
- In the sixth column, we will have signle_epithelial_size
- In the seventh column, we will have bare_nuclei
- In the eighth column, we will have bland_chromatin
- In the ninth column, we will have normal_nucleoli
- In the tenth column, we will have mitoses
- And finally, in the eleventh column, we will have class

These are factors that a pathologist would consider to determine whether or not a cell had cancer. When we discuss machine learning in healthcare, it has to be a collaborative project between doctors and computer scientists. While a doctor can help by indicating which factors are important to include, a computer scientist can help by carrying out machine learning. Now, let's move on to the next steps:

1. Since we've got the names of our columns, we will now start a DataFrame.
2. The next step will be to add pd, which stands for pandas. We're going to use the function read_csv_url, which means that the names will be equal to those listed previously.

3. Press *Shift + Enter*, and make sure that all of the imports are right.
4. We will then have to preprocess our data and carry out some visualizations, as we want to explore the dataset before we begin.

In machine learning, it's very important to understand the data that you're going to be using. This will help you pick which algorithm to use, and understand which results you're actually looking for. It is important to understand, for example, what is considered a good result, because accuracy is not always the most important classification metric. Take a look at the following steps:

1. First, our dataset contains some missing data. To deal with this, we will add a `df.replace` method.
2. If `df.replace` gives us a question mark, it means that there's no data there. We're simply going to input the value `-99999` and tell Python to ignore that data.
3. We will then perform the `print(df.axes)` operation, so that we can see the columns. We can see that we have 699 different data points, and each of those cases has 11 different columns.
4. Next, we will print the shape of the dataset using the `print(df.shape)` operation.

 We will drop the `Id` class, as we don't want to carry out machine learning on the ID column. That is because it won't tell us anything interesting.

Let's view the output of the preceding steps in the following screenshot:

```
In [4]:  # Preprocess the data
         df.replace('?',-99999, inplace=True)
         print(df.axes)

         df.drop(['id'], 1, inplace=True)

         # Print the shape of the dataset
         print(df.shape)

         [RangeIndex(start=0, stop=699, step=1), Index(['id', 'clump_thickness', 'uniform_cell_size', 'unifor
         m_cell_shape',
                 'marginal_adhesion', 'single_epithelial_size', 'bare_nuclei',
                 'bland_chromatin', 'normal_nucleoli', 'mitoses', 'class'],
                dtype='object')]
         (699, 10)
```

As we now have all of the columns, we can detect whether the tumor is benign (which means it is non-cancerous) or malignant (which means it is cancerous). We now have 10 columns, as we have dropped the ID column.

In the following screenshot, we can see the first cell in our dataset, as well as its different features:

```
In [5]:  # Do dataset visualizations
         print(df.loc[6])

         clump_thickness            1
         uniform_cell_size          1
         uniform_cell_shape         1
         marginal_adhesion          1
         single_epithelial_size     2
         bare_nuclei               10
         bland_chromatin            3
         normal_nucleoli            1
         mitoses                    1
         class                      2
         Name: 6, dtype: object
```

Now let's visualize the parameters of the dataset, in the following steps:

1. We will print the first point, so that we can see what it entails.
2. We have a value of between 0 and 10 in all of the different columns. In the class column, the number 2 represents a benign tumor, and the number 4 represents a malignant tumor. There are 699 cells in the datasets.
3. The next step will be to do a print.describe operation, which gives us the mean, standard deviation, and other aspects for each of our different parameters or features. This is shown in the following screenshot:

```
In [6]:  # Do dataset visualizations
         print(df.loc[6])
         print(df.describe())
```

```
clump_thickness           1
uniform_cell_size         1
uniform_cell_shape        1
marginal_adhesion         1
single_epithelial_size    2
bare_nuclei              10
bland_chromatin           3
normal_nucleoli           1
mitoses                   1
class                     2
Name: 6, dtype: object
       clump_thickness  uniform_cell_size  uniform_cell_shape  \
count       699.000000         699.000000          699.000000
mean          4.417740           3.134478            3.207439
std           2.815741           3.051459            2.971913
min           1.000000           1.000000            1.000000
25%           2.000000           1.000000            1.000000
50%           4.000000           1.000000            1.000000
75%           6.000000           5.000000            5.000000
max          10.000000          10.000000           10.000000

       marginal_adhesion  single_epithelial_size  bland_chromatin  \
count         699.000000              699.000000       699.000000
mean            2.806867                3.216023         3.437768
std             2.855379                2.214300         2.438364
min             1.000000                1.000000         1.000000
25%             1.000000                2.000000         2.000000
50%             1.000000                2.000000         3.000000
75%             4.000000                4.000000         5.000000
max            10.000000               10.000000        10.000000

       normal_nucleoli    mitoses       class
count       699.000000  699.000000  699.000000
mean          2.866953    1.589413    2.689557
std           3.053634    1.715078    0.951273
min           1.000000    1.000000    2.000000
25%           1.000000    1.000000    2.000000
50%           1.000000    1.000000    2.000000
75%           4.000000    1.000000    4.000000
max          10.000000   10.000000    4.000000
```

Here, we have a max value of 10 for all of the different columns, apart from the class column, which will either be 2 or 4. The mean is a little closer to 2, so we have a few more benign cases than we do malignant cases. Because the min and the max values are between 1 and 10 for all columns, it means that we've successfully ignored the missing data, so we're not factoring that in. Each column has a relatively low mean, but most of them have a max of 10, which means that we have a case where we hit 10 in all but one of the classes.

Data visualization with machine learning

Let's get started with data visualization. We will plot histograms for each variable. The steps in the preceding section are important, because we need to understand these datasets if we want to accurately and effectively use machine learning. Otherwise, we're shooting in the dark, and we might spend time on a method that doesn't need to be investigated. We will use the plt method and make a plot, in which we will add the histograms of our dataset and edit the figure sizes, to make them easier to see.

We can see the output in the following screenshot:

```
In [7]:  # Plot histograms for each variable
         df.hist(figsize = (10, 10))
         plt.show()
```

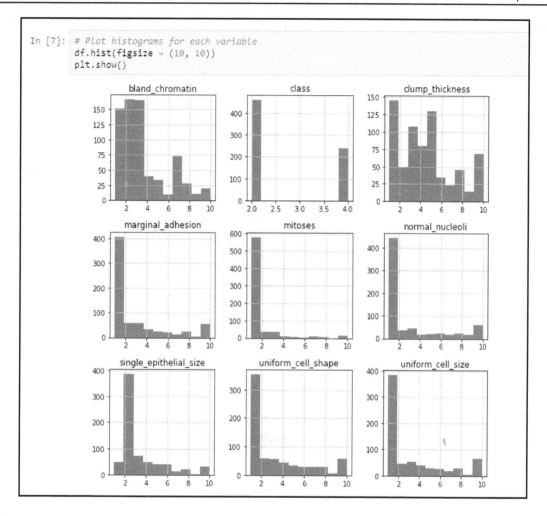

As you can see, most of the preceding histograms have the majority of their data at around 1, with some data at a slightly higher value. Each histogram, apart from `class`, has at least one case where the value is `10`. The histogram for `clump thickness` is pretty evenly distributed, while the histogram for `chromatin` is skewed to the left.

Relationships between variables

We will now look at a scatterplot matrix, to see the relationships between some of these variables. A scatterplot matrix is a very useful function to use, because it can tell us whether a linear classifier will be a good classifier for our data, or whether we have to investigate more complicated methods.

We will add a `scatter_matrix` method and adjust the size to `figsize(18, 18)`, to make it easier to see.

The output, as shown in the following screenshot, indicates the relationship between each variable and every other variable:

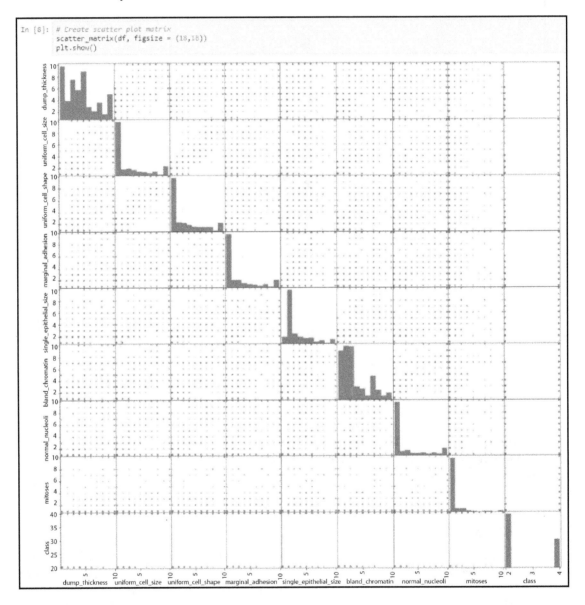

All of the variables are listed on both the x and the y axes. Where they intersect, we can see the histograms that we saw previously.

In the block indicated by the mouse cursor in the preceding screenshot, we can see that there is a pretty strong linear relationship between uniform_cell_shape and uniform_cell_size. This is expected. When we go through the preceding screenshot, we can see that some other cells have a good linear relationship. If we look at our classifications, however, there's no easy way to classify these relationships.

In class in the preceding screenshot, we can see that 4 is a malignant classification. We can also see that there are cells that are scored from 1 to 10 on clump_thickness, and were still classified as malignant.

Thus, we come to the conclusion that there aren't any strong relationships between any of the variables of our dataset.

Understanding machine learning algorithms

Since we've explored our dataset, let's take a look at how machine learning algorithms can help us to define whether a person has cancer.

The following steps will help you to better understand the machine learning algorithm:

1. The first step that we need to perform is to split our dataset into X and Y datasets for training. We won't train all of the available data, as we need to save some for our validation step. This will help us to determine how well these algorithms can generalize to new data, and not just how well they know the training data.
2. Our X data will contain all of the variables, except for the class column, and our Y data is going to be the class column, which is the classification of whether a tumor is malignant or benign.
3. Next, we will use the train_test_split function, and we will then split our data into y_train, y_test, X_train, and X_test, respectively.

4. In the same line, we will add `cross_validation.train_test_split` and `X`, `y`, `test_size`. About 20% of our data is fairly standard, so we will make the test size `0.2` to test the data as shown in the following screenshot:

```
In [9]:  # Create X and Y datasets for training
         X = np.array(df.drop(['class'], 1))
         y = np.array(df['class'])

         X_train, X_test, y_train, y_test = cross_validation.train_test_split(X, y, test_size=0.2)
```

5. Next, we will add a seed, which makes the data reproducible. We will start with a random seed, which will change the results a little bit every time.

If a seed is defined and we stay consistent, we should be able to reproduce our results.

6. In scoring, we will add `accuracy`. This is shown in the following screenshot:

```
In [10]:  # Testing Options
          seed = 8
          scoring = 'accuracy'
```

In the preceding section, you learned about how machine learning algorithms can be used for healthcare purposes. We also looked at the testing parameters that are used for this application.

Training models

Now, let's move on to actually defining the training models:

1. First, make an empty list, in which we will append the KNN model.
2. Enter the `KNeighborsClassifier` function and explore the number of neighbors.
3. Start with `n_neighbors = 5`, and play around with the variable a little, to see how it changes our results.

4. Next, we will add our models: the SVM and the SVC. We will evaluate each model, in turn.

5. The next step will be to get a results list and a names list, so that we can print out some of the information at the end.

6. We will then perform a `for` loop for each of the models defined previously, such as `name` or `model` in `models`.

7. We will also do a `k-fold` comparison, which will run each of these a couple of times, and then take the best results. The number of splits, or `n_splits`, defines how many times it runs.

8. Since we don't want a random state, we will go from the seed. Now, we will get our results. We will use the `model_selection` function that we imported previously, and the `cross_val_score`.

9. For each model, we'll provide training data to `X_train`, and then `y_train`.

10. We will also add the specification scoring, which was the `accuracy` that we added previously.

11. We will also append `results`, `name`, and we will print out a `msg`. We will then substitute some variables.

12. Finally, we will look at the mean results and the standard deviation.

13. A `k-fold` training will take place, which means that this will be run 10 times. We will receive the average result and the average accuracy for each of them. We will use a random seed of `8`, so that it is consistent across different trials and runs. Now, press *Shift + Enter*. We can see the output in the following screenshot:

```
In [11]:  # Define models to train
          models = []
          models.append(('KNN', KNeighborsClassifier(n_neighbors = 5)))
          models.append(('SVM', SVC()))

          # evaluate each model in turn
          results = []
          names = []

          for name, model in models:
              kfold = model_selection.KFold(n_splits=10, random_state = seed)
              cv_results = model_selection.cross_val_score(model, X_train, y_train, cv=kfold, scoring=scoring)
              results.append(cv_results)
              names.append(name)
              msg = "%s: %f (%f)" % (name, cv_results.mean(), cv_results.std())
              print(msg)

          KNN: 0.966039 (0.018616)
          SVM: 0.955292 (0.021477)
```

In this case, our KNN narrowly beats the SVC. We will now go back and make predictions on our validation set, because the numbers shown in the preceding screenshot just represent the accuracy of our training data. If we split up the datasets differently, we'll get the following results:

```
In [11]:  # Define models to train
          models = []
          models.append(('KNN', KNeighborsClassifier(n_neighbors = 5)))
          models.append(('SVM', SVC()))

          # evaluate each model in turn
          results = []
          names = []

          for name, model in models:
              kfold = model_selection.KFold(n_splits=10, random_state = seed)
              cv_results = model_selection.cross_val_score(model, X_train, y_train, cv=kfold, scoring=scoring)
              results.append(cv_results)
              names.append(name)
              msg = "%s: %f (%f)" % (name, cv_results.mean(), cv_results.std())
              print(msg)

          KNN: 0.966039 (0.018616)
          SVM: 0.955292 (0.021477)
```

However, once again, it looks like we have pretty similar results, at least with regard to accuracy, on the training data between our KNN and our support vector classifier. The KNN tries to cluster the different data points into two groups: malignant and benign. The SVM, on the other hand, is looking for the optimal separating hyperplane that can separate these data points into malignant cells and benign cells.

Predictions in machine learning

In this section, we will make predictions on the validation dataset. So far, machine learning hasn't been very helpful, because it has told us information about the training data that we already know. Let's have a look at the following steps:

1. First, we will make predictions on the validation sets with the y_test and the X_test that we split out earlier.
2. We'll do another for loop in for name, and model in models.
3. Then, we will do the model.fit, and it will train it once again on the X and y training data. Since we want to make predictions, we're going to use the model to actually make a prediction about the X_test data.

4. Once the model has been trained, we're going to use it to make a prediction. It will print out the `name`, the accuracy score (based on a comparison of the `y_test` data with the predictions we made), and a `classification_report`, which will tell us information about the false positives and negatives that we found.

5. Now, press *Shift + Enter*. The following screenshot shows the preceding steps, and the output:

```
In [11]:  # Make predictions on validation dataset

          for name, model in models:
              model.fit(X_train, y_train)
              predictions = model.predict(X_test)
              print(name)
              print(accuracy_score(y_test, predictions))
              print(classification_report(y_test, predictions))

          KNN
          0.9785714285714285
                          precision    recall  f1-score   support

                     2       0.98      0.99      0.98        95
                     4       0.98      0.96      0.97        45

          avg / total       0.98      0.98      0.98       140

          SVM
          0.9571428571428572
                          precision    recall  f1-score   support

                     2       1.00      0.94      0.97        95
                     4       0.88      1.00      0.94        45

          avg / total       0.96      0.96      0.96       140
```

In the preceding screenshot, we can see that the KNN got a 98% accuracy rating in the validation set. The SVM achieved a result that was a little higher, at 95%.

The preceding screenshot also shows some other measures, such as `precision`, `recall`, and the `f1-score`. The `precision` is a measure of false positives. It is actually the ratio of correctly predicted positive observations to the total predicted positive observations. A high value for `precision` means that we don't have too many false positives. The SVM has a lower precision score than the KNN, meaning that it classified a few cases as malignant when they were actually benign. It is vital to minimize the chance of getting false positives in this case, especially because we don't want to mistakenly diagnose a patient with cancer.

The `recall` is a measure of false negatives. In our KNN, we actually have a few malignant cells that are getting through our KNN without being labeled. The `f1-score` column is a combination of the `precision` and `recall` scores.

We will now go back, to do another split and randomly sort our data again. In the following screenshot, we can see that our results have changed:

```
In [11]:  # Make predictions on validation dataset

          for name, model in models:
              model.fit(X_train, y_train)
              predictions = model.predict(X_test)
              print(name)
              print(accuracy_score(y_test, predictions))
              print(classification_report(y_test, predictions))

          KNN
          0.9785714285714285
                        precision    recall  f1-score   support

                     2       0.98      0.99      0.98        95
                     4       0.98      0.96      0.97        45

          avg / total       0.98      0.98      0.98       140

          SVM
          0.9571428571428572
                        precision    recall  f1-score   support

                     2       1.00      0.94      0.97        95
                     4       0.88      1.00      0.94        45

          avg / total       0.96      0.96      0.96       140
```

This time, we did much better on both the KNN and the SVM. We also got much higher precision scores from both, at 97%. This means that we probably only got one or two false positives for our KNN. We had no false negatives for our SVM, in this case.

We will now look into another example of predicting, once again based on the cell features:

1. First, we will make an SVC and get an accuracy score for it, based on our testing data.
2. Next, we will add an example. Type in `np.array` and pick whichever data points you want. We're going to need 10 of them. We also need to remember to see whether we get a malignant prediction.
3. We will then take `example` and add `reshape` to it. We will flip it around, so that we get a column vector.
4. We will then print our prediction and press *Shift + Enter*.

The following screenshot shows that we actually did get a malignant prediction:

```
In [13]:  clf = SVC()

          clf.fit(X_train, y_train)
          accuracy = clf.score(X_test, y_test)
          print(accuracy)

          example_measures = np.array([[4,2,1,1,1,2,3,2,1]])
          example_measures = example_measures.reshape(len(example_measures), -1)
          prediction = clf.predict(example_measures)
          print(prediction)

             0.95
             [2]
```

In the preceding screenshot, we can see that we are 96% accurate, which is exactly what we were previously. By using the same model, we are actually able to predict whether a cell is malignant, based on its data.

When we run it again, we get the following results:

```
In [12]:  clf = SVC()

          clf.fit(X_train, y_train)
          accuracy = clf.score(X_test, y_test)
          print(accuracy)

          example_measures = np.array([[4,2,1,1,1,2,3,2,1]])
          example_measures = example_measures.reshape(len(example_measures), -1)
          prediction = clf.predict(example_measures)
          print(prediction)

                                                              . . .

In [13]:  clf = SVC()

          clf.fit(X_train, y_train)
          accuracy = clf.score(X_test, y_test)
          print(accuracy)

          example_measures = np.array([[4,2,1,1,1,2,3,2,1]])
          example_measures = example_measures.reshape(len(example_measures), -1)
          prediction = clf.predict(example_measures)
          print(prediction)

          0.95
          [2]
```

By changing the example from 1 to 10, the cells go from a malignant classification to a benign classification. When we change the values in the example from 4 to 5, we learn that 4 means that it is malignant. Thus, the difference between a 4 and a 5 is enough to switch our SVM from thinking it's a malignant cell to a benign cell.

Summary

In this chapter, we imported data from the UCI repository. We named the columns (or features), and then put them into a `pandas` DataFrame. We preprocessed our data and removed the ID column. We also explored the data, so that we would know more about it. We used the `describe` function, which gave us features such as the mean, the maximum, the minimum, and the different quartiles. We also created some histograms (so that we could understand the distributions of the different features) and a scatterplot matrix (so that we could look for linear relationships between the variables).

We then split our dataset up into a training set and a testing validation set. We implemented some testing parameters, built a KNN classifier and an SVC, and compared their results using a classification report. This consisted of features such as accuracy, overall accuracy, precision, recall, F1 score, and support. Finally, we built our own cell and explored what it would take to actually get a malignant or benign classification.

In the next chapter, you will learn about the detection of diabetes. Stay tuned for more!

2
Diabetes Onset Detection

The far-ranging developments in healthcare over the past few years have led to a huge collection of data that can be used for analysis. We can now easily predict the onset of various illnesses before they even happen, using a technology called **neural networks**. In this chapter, we are going to use a deep neural network and a grid search to predict the onset of diabetes for a set of patients. We will learn a lot about deep neural networks, the parameters that are used to optimize them, and how to choose the correct parameters for each.

We will cover the following topics in this chapter:

- Detecting diabetes using a deep learning grid search
- Introduction to the dataset
- Building a Keras model
- Performing a grid search using scikit-learn
- Reducing overfitting using dropout regularization
- Finding the optimal hyperparameters
- Generating predictions using optimal hyperparameters

Detecting diabetes using a grid search

We will be predicting diabetes on a of patients by using a deep learning algorithm, which we will optimize with a grid search to find the optimal hyperparameters. We are going to be doing this project in Jupyter Notebook, as follows:

1. Start by opening up Command Prompt in Windows or Terminal in Linux systems. We will navigate to our project directory using the cd command.
2. Our next step is to open the Jupyter Notebook by typing the following command:

```
jupyter notebook
```

Alternatively, you can use the `jupyter lab` command to open an instance of Jupyter Lab, which is just a better version of Notebook.

3. Once the Notebook is open, we will rename the unnamed file to `Deep Learning Grid Search`.
4. We will then import our packages using general import statements. We will print the version numbers, as shown in the following screenshot:

```
In [1]:  import sys
         import pandas
         import numpy
         import sklearn
         import keras

         print('Python: {}'.format(sys.version))
         print('Pandas: {}'.format(pandas.__version__))
         print('Numpy: {}'.format(numpy.__version__))
         print('Sklearn: {}'.format(sklearn.__version__))
         print('Keras: {}'.format(keras.__version__))

         C:\ProgramData\Anaconda3\lib\site-packages\h5py\__init__.py:36: FutureWarning: Conversion of the
         p.dtype(float).type`.
           from ._conv import register_converters as _register_converters
         Using TensorFlow backend.
         Python: 3.6.5 |Anaconda, Inc.| (default, Mar 29 2018, 13:32:41) [MSC v.1900 64 bit (AMD64)]
         Pandas: 0.23.0
         Numpy: 1.14.3
         Sklearn: 0.19.1
         Keras: 2.2.2
```

Keras has two options: TensorFlow and Theano. These are both deep learning packages, but we will be using Theano in this chapter. To switch from TensorFlow to Theano, perform the following steps:

1. Go to the `.keras` folder that is present in the Windows `Users` folder. We can navigate to this folder using `C:|Users|<yourusername>|.keras`. This folder contains a `datasets` folder and `keras.json` file, as shown in the following screenshot:

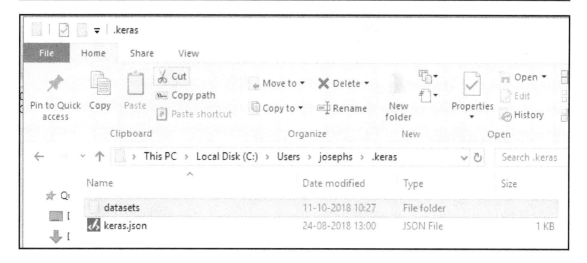

If you open up the `keras.json` file in Notepad, you'll see the following details:

```
keras.json - Notepad
File   Edit   Format   View   Help
{
     "floatx": "float32",
     "epsilon": 1e-07,
     "backend": "tensorflow",
     "image_data_format": "channels_last"
}
```

In the preceding screenshot, we can see that Keras is currently using the TensorFlow backend.

2. Since we will be using Theano, change the `backend` variable to `theano`. We are now all set to continue.

 If you were using TensorFlow previously, you might have to install Theano first.

We will now change the naming convention for `pandas` and `numpy`, so that we can use their abbreviated terms in the future. This can be done using the following lines of code:

```
import pandas as pd
import numpy as np
```

Introduction to the dataset

Our next step is to import the Pima Indians diabetes dataset, which contains the details of about 750 patients:

1. The dataset that we need can be found at `https://raw.githubusercontent.com/ jbrownlee/Datasets/master/pima-indians-diabetes.data.csv`. We can import it by using the following line:

   ```
   url =
   "https://raw.githubusercontent.com/jbrownlee/Datasets/master/pima-i
   ndians-diabetes.data.csv"
   ```

2. If we navigate to the preceding URL, we can see a lot of raw information. Once we have imported the dataset, we have to define column names. We will do this using the following lines of code:

   ```
   names = ['n_pregnant', 'glucose_concentration', 'blood_pressure (mm
   Hg)', 'skin_thickness (mm)', 'serum_insulin (mu U/ml)', 'BMI',
   'pedigree_function', 'age', 'class']
   ```

   As can be seen in the preceding code block, we have several parameters, including `blood_pressure`, `age`, and `BMI`.

3. Once we have defined the names of the columns, we have to read all the data into a `pandas` DataFrame. Since our dataset is in CSV format, we can use the `pd.read_csv()` function to do this, as shown in the following screenshot:

```
In [2]: import pandas as pd
        import numpy as np

        # import the uci pima indians diabetes dataset
        url = "https://raw.githubusercontent.com/jbrownlee/Datasets/master/pima-indians-diabetes.data.csv"
        names = ['n_pregnant', 'glucose_concentration', 'blood_pressure (mm Hg)', 'skin_thickness (mm)', 'serum_insulin (mu U/ml)',
                 'BMI', 'pedigree_function', 'age', 'class']
        df = pd.read_csv(url, names = names)
```

4. We will now have a look at the dataset by using the `describe()` function, as shown in the following screenshot:

```
In [3]:  # Describe the dataset
         df.describe()
```

Out[3]:

	n_pregnant	glucose_concentration	blood_pressure (mm Hg)	skin_thickness (mm)	serum_insulin (mu U/ml)	BMI	pedigree_function	age	class
count	768.000000	768.000000	768.000000	768.000000	768.000000	768.000000	768.000000	768.000000	768.000000
mean	3.845052	120.894531	69.105469	20.536458	79.799479	31.992578	0.471876	33.240885	0.348958
std	3.369578	31.972618	19.355807	15.952218	115.244002	7.884160	0.331329	11.760232	0.476951
min	0.000000	0.000000	0.000000	0.000000	0.000000	0.000000	0.078000	21.000000	0.000000
25%	1.000000	99.000000	62.000000	0.000000	0.000000	27.300000	0.243750	24.000000	0.000000
50%	3.000000	117.000000	72.000000	23.000000	30.500000	32.000000	0.372500	29.000000	0.000000
75%	6.000000	140.250000	80.000000	32.000000	127.250000	36.600000	0.626250	41.000000	1.000000
max	17.000000	199.000000	122.000000	99.000000	846.000000	67.100000	2.420000	81.000000	1.000000

As shown in the preceding screenshot, we have 8 columns and `768` instances for each column. This DataFrame gives us various measures for each column, including `mean`, `min`, `std`, and `max`. `n_pregnant`, for example, goes all the way from 0 to somebody who was pregnant 17 times, which is the maximum value. However, in most of the columns, we notice that there are quite a few places where the value is zero, which may represent missing data.

Having missing data will throw off our algorithm's accuracy. Let's deal with this first.

Preprocessing the dataset

Since we have missing data values, we will have to sort through the data to understand what's going on:

1. To do this, we will use the following code snippet to pull up a DataFrame where the glucose concentration of a patient is listed as 0:

   ```
   df[df['glucose_concentration'] == 0]
   ```

   This provides us with a DataFrame, as seen in the following screenshot:

```
In [4]:  df[df['glucose_concentration'] == 0]
```

Out[4]:

	n_pregnant	glucose_concentration	blood_pressure (mm Hg)	skin_thickness (mm)	serum_insulin (mu U/ml)	BMI	pedigree_function	age	class
75	1	0	48	20	0	24.7	0.140	22	0
182	1	0	74	20	23	27.7	0.299	21	0
342	1	0	68	35	0	32.0	0.389	22	0
349	5	0	80	32	0	41.0	0.346	37	1
502	6	0	68	41	0	39.0	0.727	41	1

Here, we can see that there are five cases where the `glucose_concentration` is 0, meaning that it is likely that there is some missing information in the dataset. This will hinder the accuracy of our algorithm, so we have to preprocess the data.

2. We're going to mark the missing values as `NaN`, and drop them. To do this, we're going to define the columns we want to look at. We will define all of the columns, excluding those for `n_pregnancy`, `age`, and `class`. This can be done as follows:

```
columns = ['glucose_concentration', 'blood_pressure (mm Hg)',
    'skin_thickness (mm)', 'serum_insulin (mu U/ml)', 'BMI']
```

3. After defining the columns, we have to replace all the zero values with `NaN`. This can be done as follows:

```
for col in columns:
    df[col].replace(0, np.NaN, inplace=True)
```

4. We will then take another look at the DataFrame to ensure that the preceding commands have worked. We can do this with the `describe()` function, as shown in the following screenshot:

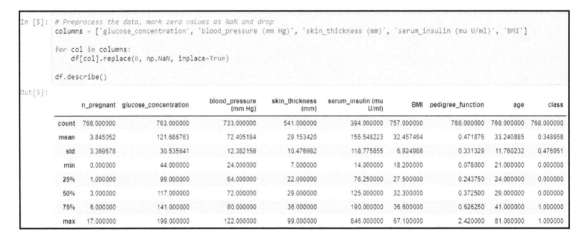

```
In [5]:  # Preprocess the data, mark zero values as NaN and drop
         columns = ['glucose_concentration', 'blood_pressure (mm Hg)', 'skin_thickness (mm)', 'serum_insulin (mu U/ml)', 'BMI']

         for col in columns:
             df[col].replace(0, np.NaN, inplace=True)

         df.describe()
```

Out[5]:

	n_pregnant	glucose_concentration	blood_pressure (mm Hg)	skin_thickness (mm)	serum_insulin (mu U/ml)	BMI	pedigree_function	age	class
count	768.000000	763.000000	733.000000	541.000000	394.000000	757.000000	768.000000	768.000000	768.000000
mean	3.845052	121.686763	72.405184	29.153420	155.548223	32.457464	0.471876	33.240885	0.348958
std	3.369578	30.535641	12.382158	10.476982	118.775855	6.924988	0.331329	11.760232	0.476951
min	0.000000	44.000000	24.000000	7.000000	14.000000	18.200000	0.078000	21.000000	0.000000
25%	1.000000	99.000000	64.000000	22.000000	76.250000	27.500000	0.243750	24.000000	0.000000
50%	3.000000	117.000000	72.000000	29.000000	125.000000	32.300000	0.372500	29.000000	0.000000
75%	6.000000	141.000000	80.000000	36.000000	190.000000	36.600000	0.626250	41.000000	1.000000
max	17.000000	199.000000	122.000000	99.000000	846.000000	67.100000	2.420000	81.000000	1.000000

We can now see that there are a number of instances in the columns modified by us that show some changes. For example, the number of instances in `serum_insulin` has dropped to `394`, from the initial `768`.

5. Now that we know which columns have rows with missing values, we can drop the missing values and print the DataFrame again. This can be done as follows:

```
df.dropna(inplace=True)
df.describe()
```

This will give us an updated DataFrame without any missing values, as shown in the following screenshot:

```
In [6]: # Drop rows with missing values
        df.dropna(inplace=True)

        # summarize the number of rows and columns in df
        df.describe()
```

Out[6]:

	n_pregnant	glucose_concentration	blood_pressure (mm Hg)	skin_thickness (mm)	serum_insulin (mu U/ml)	BMI	pedigree_function	age	class
count	392.000000	392.000000	392.000000	392.000000	392.000000	392.000000	392.000000	392.000000	392.000000
mean	3.301020	122.627551	70.663265	29.145408	156.056122	33.086224	0.523046	30.864796	0.331633
std	3.211424	30.860781	12.496092	10.516424	118.841690	7.027659	0.345488	10.200777	0.471401
min	0.000000	56.000000	24.000000	7.000000	14.000000	18.200000	0.085000	21.000000	0.000000
25%	1.000000	99.000000	62.000000	21.000000	76.750000	28.400000	0.269750	23.000000	0.000000
50%	2.000000	119.000000	70.000000	29.000000	125.500000	33.200000	0.449500	27.000000	0.000000
75%	5.000000	143.000000	78.000000	37.000000	190.000000	37.100000	0.687000	36.000000	1.000000
max	17.000000	198.000000	110.000000	63.000000	846.000000	67.100000	2.420000	81.000000	1.000000

We were able to drop every row that had a missing value, so we now only have 392 instances.

6. Let's go ahead and convert this dataset into a NumPy array. This can be done using the `df.values()` function. Once we have done this, we have to print the DataFrame shape to check whether everything has been converted correctly. This is shown in the following screenshot:

```
In [8]: # Convert dataframe to numpy array
        dataset = df.values
        print(dataset.shape)

        (392, 9)
```

We can see that we have 392 patients and 9 columns for each patient.

7. Let's split this into two sets: an input, X, and an output, Y. NumPy arrays are really easy to index. We will split the dataset using the following lines of code:

```
X = dataset[:, 0:8]
Y = dataset[:, 8].astype(int)
```

8. We also have to add `.astype(int)` to let the application know that the values are all integers.

9. Once we have split the dataset, we will print the `X.shape`, the `Y.shape`, and the first five instances of X just to see whether everything is running smoothly. The output that we get after printing will look similar to the following screenshot:

```
In [17]:  print(X.shape)
          print(Y.shape)
          print(X[:5])

(392, 8)
(392,)
[[1.000e+00 8.900e+01 6.600e+01 2.300e+01 9.400e+01 2.810e+01 1.670e-01
  2.100e+01]
 [0.000e+00 1.370e+02 4.000e+01 3.500e+01 1.680e+02 4.310e+01 2.288e+00
  3.300e+01]
 [3.000e+00 7.800e+01 5.000e+01 3.200e+01 8.800e+01 3.100e+01 2.480e-01
  2.600e+01]
 [2.000e+00 1.970e+02 7.000e+01 4.500e+01 5.430e+02 3.050e+01 1.580e-01
  5.300e+01]
 [1.000e+00 1.890e+02 6.000e+01 2.300e+01 8.460e+02 3.010e+01 3.980e-01
  5.900e+01]]
```

In the preceding screenshot, we can see that our first five X values are all floats. If we print the Y values, we get integers.

Normalizing the dataset

Before we go any further, we need to normalize the information so that the algorithm can read the data consistently:

1. Let's normalize the data using the `StandardScaler` from the `sklearn` library. We will import the required tools and fit the data to the `scaler` using the following lines of code:

```
from sklearn.preprocessing import StandardScaler
scaler = StandardScaler().fit(X)
```

If we print this `scaler`, we will get the following output:

```
In [12]: print(scaler)
         StandardScaler(copy=True, with_mean=True, with_std=True)
```

Here, we've created a matrix that will do the scaling for us. There are a few different parameters that can be used to scale each of our different columns.

First, however, we have to transform and display the training data. We will do that using the code shown in the following screenshot:

```
In [13]: # Transform and display the training data
         X_standardized = scaler.transform(X)

         data = pd.DataFrame(X_standardized)
         data.describe()
```

Out[13]:		0	1	2	3	4	5	6	7
	count	3.920000e+02	3.920000e+02	3.920000e+02	3.920000e+02	3.920000e+02	3.920000e+02	3.920000e+02	3.920000e+02
	mean	-4.021726e-17	3.129583e-17	-4.641624e-16	1.042250e-16	6.485742e-17	1.543550e-16	3.880116e-17	1.028089e-16
	std	1.001278e+00	1.001278e+00	1.001278e+00	1.001278e+00	1.001278e+00	1.001278e+00	1.001278e+00	1.001278e+00
	min	-1.029213e+00	-2.161731e+00	-3.739001e+00	-2.108484e+00	-1.196867e+00	-2.120941e+00	-1.269525e+00	-9.682991e-01
	25%	-7.174265e-01	-7.665958e-01	-6.941640e-01	-7.755315e-01	-6.681786e-01	-6.676780e-01	-7.340909e-01	-7.719850e-01
	50%	-4.056403e-01	-1.176959e-01	-5.314565e-02	-1.384444e-02	-2.574448e-01	1.621036e-02	-2.131475e-01	-3.793569e-01
	75%	5.297185e-01	6.609841e-01	5.878727e-01	7.478426e-01	2.859877e-01	5.718696e-01	4.751644e-01	5.040564e-01
	max	4.271153e+00	2.445459e+00	3.151946e+00	3.223325e+00	5.812990e+00	4.846172e+00	5.497667e+00	4.921123e+00

Here, we still have 392 instances, but they have essentially been normalized so that they have a mean of nearly zero and a standard deviation of nearly 1. All of our parameters now are on an equal footing, and won't be weighted inappropriately by the machine learning algorithm that we are going to develop. The dataset is now all set up and ready to go.

Building our Keras model

We'll now start building our Keras model, which is a deep learning algorithm:

1. The first thing that we're going to do is import the necessary packages and layers. We will do that by running the following lines of code:

```
from sklearn.model_selection import GridSearchCV, KFold
from keras.models import Sequential
from keras.layers import Dense
from keras.wrappers.scikit_learn import KerasClassifier
from keras.optimizers import Adam
```

In the preceding code snippet , `GridSearchCV` is the function we will use to perform a grid search, and `KFold` will be used for performing the k-fold cross-validation. `KerasClassifier` is used as the wrapper. `Adam` is the optimizer that we will be using for this model; the rest of the functions are all general functions used to define the model:

2. Let's start by defining the model. We will use a `create_model()` function, because we have to repeatedly reinitialize our model.
3. The first thing to do is define the type of model. In our case, this will be `Sequential`.
4. After this, we have to add the following layers to the model:

- The input layer, which is the first layer
- A dense layer, where all the neurons are connected to every input
- The output layer, which is the last layer

Since we want to create a deep learning model, we also have to create multiple hidden layers. A hidden layer comes between the input and the output layer.

5. Let's now compile the model. We will start by defining our optimizer, which is the `Adam` optimizer, and we will set a base learning rate of 0.01. This controls how fast you want the parameters of your model to be updated. The whole process of defining our model can be done using the following lines of code:

```
def create_model():
    # create model
    model = Sequential()
    model.add(Dense(8, input_dim = 8, kernel_initializer='normal',
activation='relu'))
    model.add(Dense(4, input_dim = 8, kernel_initializer='normal',
activation='relu'))
```

```
model.add(Dense(1, activation='sigmoid'))

# compile the model
adam = Adam(lr = 0.01)
model.compile(loss = 'binary_crossentropy', optimizer = adam,
metrics = ['accuracy'])
return model
```

In the preceding code snippet, we have initialized and compiled a model. We will get the following output when we print the model characteristics:

```
In [15]:  # Start defining the model
          def create_model():
              # create model
              model = Sequential()
              model.add(Dense(8, input_dim = 8, kernel_initializer='normal', activation='relu'))
              model.add(Dense(4, input_dim = 8, kernel_initializer='normal', activation='relu'))
              model.add(Dense(1, activation='sigmoid'))

              # compile the model
              adam = Adam(lr = 0.01)
              model.compile(loss = 'binary_crossentropy', optimizer = adam, metrics = ['accuracy'])
              return model

          model = create_model()
          print(model.summary())

          _____
          Layer (type)                 Output Shape              Param #
          =================================================================
          dense_1 (Dense)              (None, 8)                 72
          _____
          dense_2 (Dense)              (None, 4)                 36
          _____
          dense_3 (Dense)              (None, 1)                 5
          =================================================================
          Total params: 113
          Trainable params: 113
          Non-trainable params: 0
          _____
          None
```

As we can see in the preceding screenshot, we have all the information for each layer. The total number of parameters in this network is 113, so it's a relatively small network. This gives us some helpful information about our network.

Performing a grid search using scikit-learn

It's now time to prepare our grid search algorithm. We will follow a step-by-step process to make it easier to understand and execute:

1. The first thing that we will do is copy the `create_model()` function, which we created in the *Building a Keras model* section, and paste it into a new cell, as shown in the following screenshot:

```
In [16]:
    def create_model():
        # create model
        model = Sequential()
        model.add(Dense(8, input_dim = 8, kernel_initializer='normal', activation='relu'))
        model.add(Dense(4, input_dim = 8, kernel_initializer='normal', activation='relu'))
        model.add(Dense(1, activation='sigmoid'))

        # compile the model
        adam = Adam(lr = 0.01)
        model.compile(loss = 'binary_crossentropy', optimizer = adam, metrics = ['accuracy'])
        return model
```

2. Now, we will define a random seed through NumPy. This helps us to create results that are reproducible. We are also going to add random initialization of weights and random divisions of data into different groups. We will set a starting point so that we have the same initialization and the same divisions for all the data. This can be done by adding a few lines of code above the `create_model()` function, as shown in the following screenshot:

```
In [16]:   # Define a random seed
           seed = 6
           np.random.seed(seed)

           # Start defining the model
           def create_model():
               # create model
               model = Sequential()
               model.add(Dense(8, input_dim = 8, kernel_initializer='normal', activation='relu'))
               model.add(Dense(4, input_dim = 8, kernel_initializer='normal', activation='relu'))
               model.add(Dense(1, activation='sigmoid'))

               # compile the model
               adam = Adam(lr = 0.01)
               model.compile(loss = 'binary_crossentropy', optimizer = adam, metrics = ['accuracy'])
               return model
```

3. Our next step is to initialize the `KerasClassifier` that we imported in the early stages. This is done by using the following line after the `create_model()` function:

```
model = KerasClassifier(build_fn = create_model, verbose = 0)
```

We can see two parameters present in the function in the preceding code block. The first one is `build_fn`, which defines how we're going to build our models. The second one is `verbose`, which controls how much information is going to print when we run the cell. We're going to set this to `0`.

If we want to see the algorithm at work, we can set the verbose function to `1`.

4. We now have to define the grid search parameters so that our model knows what it's trying to optimize. To do this, we simply define the `batch_size` variable by assigning values of `[10,20,40]` to it. The `batch_size` variable refers to the number of steps that the model should take, or the number of inputs it should look at, before it sums all the changes to the gradients and updates the weight parameters. The `epochs` parameter defines how long we train the network. We will define this as `[10,50,100]`.

5. However, for the grid search algorithm to work, we have to turn these parameters into a dictionary by using the `dict()` command. The following line shows the command and the parameters used:

```
param_grid = dict(batch_size=batch_size, epochs=epochs)
```

So far, our code should look similar to the following screenshot:

```
In [19]:  # Define a random seed
          seed = 6
          np.random.seed(seed)

          # Start defining the model
          def create_model():
              # create model
              model = Sequential()
              model.add(Dense(8, input_dim = 8, kernel_initializer='normal', activation='relu'))
              model.add(Dense(4, input_dim = 8, kernel_initializer='normal', activation='relu'))
              model.add(Dense(1, activation='sigmoid'))

              # compile the model
              adam = Adam(lr = 0.01)
              model.compile(loss = 'binary_crossentropy', optimizer = adam, metrics = ['accuracy'])
              return model

          # create the model
          model = KerasClassifier(build_fn = create_model, verbose = 0)

          # define the grid search parameters
          batch_size = [10, 20, 40]
          epochs = [10, 50, 100]

          # make a dictionary of the grid search parameters
          param_grid = dict(batch_size=batch_size, epochs=epochs)
```

6. We will now build and fit the grid search. This is where we will be doing our hyperparameter optimization. We're going to define our grid and initiate the GridSearchCV class instance, which comes with a lot of parameters. After that, we have to fit the data to our instance. This is done as follows:

```
grid = GridSearchCV(estimator = model, param_grid = param_grid, cv
= KFold(random_state=seed), verbose = 10)
grid_results = grid.fit(X_standardized, Y)
```

In the preceding code snippet, we can see a lot of parameters:

- The estimator parameter indicates which model to use.
- The param_grid parameter defines the parameter grid.
- We define cross-validation as cv. In our case, this will be k-fold cross-validation. This will divide the dataset into a certain number of different sets. We're going to be doing three-fold cross-validation, so our dataset will be split into three parts. Two of these parts are going to go into the training data, while the third part will be reserved for the validation test set. K-fold cross-validation will switch which third of the data it uses for testing each time. It'll run each network three times, and each example will be used in the test set once.
- The verbose parameter has been set to 0, so that we will see only the final output.

Let's summarize the results, so that we can read them easily:

```
print("Best: {0}, using {1}".format(grid_results.best_score_,
grid_results.best_params_))
means = grid_results.cv_results_['mean_test_score']
stds = grid_result.cv_results_['std_test_score']
params = grid_results.cv_results_['params']
for mean, stdev, param in zip(means, stds, params):
    print('{0} ({1}) with: {2}'.format(mean, stdev, param))
```

7. It's now time to run the search and see the results. First, let's recap our grid search cell by comparing it to the following screenshot:

```
In [11]:  # Do a grid search for the optimal batch size and number of epochs
          # Define a random seed
          seed = 6
          np.random.seed(seed)

          # Start defining the model
          def create_model():
              # create model
              model = Sequential()
              model.add(Dense(8, input_dim = 8, kernel_initializer='normal', activation='relu'))
              model.add(Dense(4, input_dim = 8, kernel_initializer='normal', activation='relu'))
              model.add(Dense(1, activation='sigmoid'))

              # compile the model
              adam = Adam(lr = 0.01)
              model.compile(loss = 'binary_crossentropy', optimizer = adam, metrics = ['accuracy'])
              return model

          # create the model
          model = KerasClassifier(build_fn = create_model, verbose = 0)

          # define the grid search parameters
          batch_size = [10, 20, 40]
          epochs = [10, 50, 100]

          # make a dictionary of the grid search parameters
          param_grid = dict(batch_size=batch_size, epochs=epochs)

          # build and fit the GridSearchCV
          grid = GridSearchCV(estimator = model, param_grid = param_grid, cv = KFold(random_state=seed), verbose = 10)
          grid_results = grid.fit(X_standardized, Y)

          # summarize the results
          print("Best: {0}, using {1}".format(grid_results.best_score_, grid_results.best_params_))
          means = grid_results.cv_results_['mean_test_score']
          stds = grid_results.cv_results_['std_test_score']
          params = grid_results.cv_results_['params']
          for mean, stdev, param in zip(means, stds, params):
              print('{0} ({1}) with: {2}'.format(mean, stdev, param))
```

After running the cell, we get the following output:

```
Fitting 3 folds for each of 9 candidates, totalling 27 fits
[CV] batch_size=10, epochs=10 ..............................        [CV] batch_size=20, epochs=50 ..............................
[CV]  batch_size=10, epochs=10, score=0.7480915975934677, total=   9.6s   [CV]  batch_size=20, epochs=50, score=0.8000000165059016, total=  10.1s
[CV] batch_size=10, epochs=10 ..............................        [CV] batch_size=20, epochs=100 .............................
[Parallel(n_jobs=1)]: Done   1 out of   1 | elapsed:    9.7s remaining:    0.0s   [CV]  batch_size=20, epochs=100, score=0.7480915594863484, total=  12.7s
[CV]  batch_size=10, epochs=10, score=0.7633587722559921, total=   7.2s   [CV] batch_size=20, epochs=100 .............................
[CV] batch_size=10, epochs=10 ..............................        [CV]  batch_size=20, epochs=100, score=0.7862595486096922, total=  14.3s
[Parallel(n_jobs=1)]: Done   2 out of   2 | elapsed:   17.0s remaining:    0.0s   [CV] batch_size=20, epochs=100 .............................
[CV]  batch_size=10, epochs=10, score=0.8230769175740958, total=   6.6s   [CV]  batch_size=20, epochs=100, score=0.8230769359148465, total=  12.7s
[CV] batch_size=10, epochs=50 ..............................        [CV] batch_size=40, epochs=10 ..............................
[Parallel(n_jobs=1)]: Done   3 out of   3 | elapsed:   23.7s remaining:    0.0s   [CV]  batch_size=40, epochs=10, score=0.7175572364384891, total=   8.0s
[CV] batch_size=10, epochs=50 ..............................        [CV] batch_size=40, epochs=10 ..............................
[CV]  batch_size=10, epochs=50, score=0.7175572619183372, total=  55.7s   [CV]  batch_size=40, epochs=10, score=0.7709923614672436, total=   7.3s
[CV] batch_size=10, epochs=50 ..............................        [CV] batch_size=40, epochs=10 ..............................
[Parallel(n_jobs=1)]: Done   4 out of   4 | elapsed:    1.3min remaining:    0.0s   [CV]  batch_size=40, epochs=10, score=0.8230769313298739, total=   7.2s
[CV]  batch_size=10, epochs=50, score=0.7328244229309432, total=  14.4s   [CV] batch_size=40, epochs=50 ..............................
[CV] batch_size=10, epochs=50 ..............................        [CV]  batch_size=40, epochs=50, score=0.7480916048734243, total=   8.1s
[Parallel(n_jobs=1)]: Done   5 out of   5 | elapsed:    1.6min remaining:    0.0s   [CV] batch_size=40, epochs=50 ..............................
[CV]  batch_size=10, epochs=50, score=0.8153846128336318, total=  14.5s   [CV]  batch_size=40, epochs=50, score=0.7938931293159951, total=   8.5s
[CV] batch_size=10, epochs=100 .............................        [CV] batch_size=40, epochs=50 ..............................
[Parallel(n_jobs=1)]: Done   6 out of   6 | elapsed:    1.8min remaining:    0.0s   [CV]  batch_size=40, epochs=50, score=0.8307692179313073, total=   8.3s
[CV]  batch_size=10, epochs=100, score=0.7251908469748131, total=  17.2s   [CV] batch_size=40, epochs=100 .............................
[CV] batch_size=10, epochs=100 .............................        [CV]  batch_size=40, epochs=100, score=0.7175572546383607, total=   9.8s
[Parallel(n_jobs=1)]: Done   7 out of   7 | elapsed:    2.1min remaining:    0.0s   [CV] batch_size=40, epochs=100 .............................
[CV]  batch_size=10, epochs=100, score=0.7328244297559825, total=  15.1s   [CV]  batch_size=40, epochs=100, score=0.7709923695971947, total=   9.7s
[CV] batch_size=10, epochs=100 .............................        [CV] batch_size=40, epochs=100 .............................
[Parallel(n_jobs=1)]: Done   8 out of   8 | elapsed:    2.4min remaining:    0.0s   [CV]  batch_size=40, epochs=100, score=0.7999999998166011, total=   9.6s
[CV]  batch_size=10, epochs=100, score=0.8153846080466591, total=  15.4s   [Parallel(n_jobs=1)]: Done  27 out of  27 | elapsed:    5.8min finished
[Parallel(n_jobs=1)]: Done   9 out of   9 | elapsed:    2.6min remaining:    0.0s   Best: 0.7998163227292956, using {'batch_size': 40, 'epochs': 50}
[CV] batch_size=20, epochs=10 ..............................        0.7780612187117947 (0.0323174727192797) with: {'batch_size': 10, 'epochs': 10}
[CV]  batch_size=20, epochs=10, score=0.7251908351448836, total=   8.2s   0.7551020417286425 (0.0429103522102097) with: {'batch_size': 10, 'epochs': 50}
[CV] batch_size=20, epochs=10 ..............................        0.7576530619847531 (0.0407657977678057) with: {'batch_size': 10, 'epochs': 100}
[CV]  batch_size=20, epochs=10, score=0.7709923695971947, total=   8.7s   0.7653061229051376 (0.0307857193119481906) with: {'batch_size': 20, 'epochs': 10}
[CV] batch_size=20, epochs=10 ..............................        0.7755102118363186 (0.0183448390150440526) with: {'batch_size': 20, 'epochs': 50}
[CV]  batch_size=20, epochs=10, score=0.8000000027509836, total=  11.3s   0.7857142895156023 (0.0365953219092261793) with: {'batch_size': 20, 'epochs': 100}
[CV] batch_size=20, epochs=50 ..............................        0.7764981591598841 (0.043052426411003683) with: {'batch_size': 40, 'epochs': 10}
[CV]  batch_size=20, epochs=50, score=0.755725184697326, total=   9.6s   0.7908163227292956 (0.0338015720820859) with: {'batch_size': 40, 'epochs': 50}
[CV] batch_size=20, epochs=50 ..............................        0.7627551034892903 (0.0341378931539789) with: {'batch_size': 40, 'epochs': 100}
[CV]  batch_size=20, epochs=50, score=0.7789923796071351, total=   9.7s
```

We're getting a pretty high accuracy of almost 88% on our training set. On our testing set, however, we only have 77.8% accuracy, which shows that our model can't generalize well to new data. We might be overfitting our training data a bit too heavily in this particular case. 79.33% is the best accuracy we can achieve on our testing dataset, using 100 epochs with a batch size of 20. Since we're trying to predict whether an individual has diabetes, even having an accuracy rate that is 2% higher will be very valuable. We were able to obtain this increase simply by optimizing the batch size and epochs.

Reducing overfitting using dropout regularization

We will now use the information we gained in the *Performing a grid search using scikit-learn* section to optimize other aspects of our model. It looks like we might be overfitting the data a little bit, as we are getting better results on our training data than our testing data. We're now going to look at adding in dropout regularization:

1. Our first step is to copy the code that is present in the grid search cell that we ran in the previous section, and paste it in a fresh cell. We will keep the general structure of the code and play around with some of the parameters present.

2. We will then import the `Dropout` function from `keras.layers` using the following line:

```
from keras.layers import Dropout
```

3. We will now convert the learning rate into a variable by defining it in the `Adam` optimizer code block. We will use `learn_rate` as the variable. Our code will now look as follows:

```
In [15]:   # Do a grid search for the optimal batch size and number of epochs
           from keras.layers import Dropout

           # Define a random seed
           seed = 6
           np.random.seed(seed)

           # Start defining the model
           def create_model():
               # create model
               model = Sequential()
               model.add(Dense(8, input_dim = 8, kernel_initializer='normal', activation='relu'))
               model.add(Dense(4, input_dim = 8, kernel_initializer='normal', activation='relu'))
               model.add(Dense(1, activation='sigmoid'))

               # compile the model
               adam = Adam(lr = learn_rate)
               model.compile(loss = 'binary_crossentropy', optimizer = adam, metrics = ['accuracy'])
               return model

           # create the model
           model = KerasClassifier(build_fn = create_model, verbose = 0)

           # define the grid search parameters
           batch_size = [10, 20, 40]
           epochs = [10, 50, 100]

           # make a dictionary of the grid search parameters
           param_grid = dict(batch_size=batch_size, epochs=epochs)

           # build and fit the GridSearchCV
           grid = GridSearchCV(estimator = model, param_grid = param_grid, cv = KFold(random_state=seed), verbose = 10)
           grid_results = grid.fit(X_standardized, Y)

           # summarize the results
           print("Best: {0}, using {1}".format(grid_results.best_score_, grid_results.best_params_))
           means = grid_results.cv_results_['mean_test_score']
           stds = grid_results.cv_results_['std_test_score']
           params = grid_results.cv_results_['params']
           for mean, stdev, param in zip(means, stds, params):
               print('{0} ({1}) with: {2}'.format(mean, stdev, param))
```

4. Now, we will add the `learn_rate` and `dropout_rate` variables to the `create_model()` function, since we have to call these variables every time we run the function. Our `create_model()` function now becomes `create_model (learn_rate, dropout_rate)`.

5. Our next step is to add a `Dropout` layer between the input, output, and hidden layers. Our `create_model()` function will now look as follows:

```
# Start defining the model
def create_model(learn_rate, dropout_rate):
    # create model
    model = Sequential()
    model.add(Dense(8, input_dim = 8, kernel_initializer='normal', activation='relu'))
    model.add(Dropout(dropout_rate))
    model.add(Dense(4, input_dim = 8, kernel_initializer='normal', activation='relu'))
    model.add(Dropout(dropout_rate))
    model.add(Dense(1, activation='sigmoid'))
```

In the preceding screenshot, the `Dropout` layer periodically knocks out some of the neurons so that the others have to pick up the slack. As a result, it prevents any one neuron from becoming too important to the overall network, or too heavily weighted. This is going to help our network generalize to new models more effectively.

6. We will now modify the `KerasClassifier` a little because we know that the best scenario is to have a batch size of 20 with 100 epochs. We will do this by adding a couple of parameters to the `KerasClassifier`, as shown in the following screenshot:

```
# create the model
model = KerasClassifier(build_fn = create_model, epochs = 100, batch_size = 20, verbose = 0)
```

7. We will now go to our grid search parameters and define the learn rates that we want in this scenario. These will be `0.001`, `0.01`, and `0.1`. We will also define our `dropout_rate` as `0.0`, `0.1`, and `0.2`. Our grid search parameters will now look as follows:

```
# define the grid search parameters
learn_rate = [0.001, 0.01, 0.1]
dropout_rate = [0.0, 0.1, 0.2]
```

The learn rate will control how fast we update the parameters of our networks. If the changes made to the weights are too large, the algorithm may bounce around and it will never find the local minima in the loss or in the accuracy. On the other hand, if the learning rate is too large, we won't update the parameters frequently enough to get to a good stopping criterion, or the accuracy that we desire. However, the dropout rate is a regularization technique to improve our model's ability to generalize to new data.

8. We will now make a dictionary of the grid search parameters for this model by assigning the `learn_rate` and the `dropout_rate` variables, as shown in the following screenshot:

```
# make a dictionary of the grid search parameters
param_grid = dict(learn_rate=learn_rate, dropout_rate=dropout_rate)
```

9. We are now ready to execute the modified grid search. First, let's recap all the changes that we have made to the code:

```
# import necessary packages
from keras.layers import Dropout          # Added this import line

# Define a random seed
seed = 6
np.random.seed(seed)

# Start defining the model
def create_model(learn_rate, dropout_rate): # Added the learn rate
and dropout variables
    # create model
    model = Sequential()
    model.add(Dense(8, input_dim = 8, kernel_initializer='normal',
activation='relu'))
    model.add(Dropout(dropout_rate))        # Added a Dropout layer
```

```
here
    model.add(Dense(4, input_dim = 8, kernel_initializer='normal',
activation='relu'))
    model.add(Dropout(dropout_rate))          # Added a Dropout layer
here
    model.add(Dense(1, activation='sigmoid'))
    # compile the model
    adam = Adam(lr = learn_rate)              # Defined the
learn_rate variable here
    model.compile(loss = 'binary_crossentropy', optimizer = adam,
metrics = ['accuracy'])
    return model

# create the model
# Defined 2 parameters here
model = KerasClassifier(build_fn = create_model, epochs = 100,
batch_size = 20, verbose = 0)

# Defined the grid search parameters here
learn_rate = [0.001, 0.01, 0.1]
dropout_rate = [0.0, 0.1, 0.2]

# Made a dictionary of the grid search parameters here
param_grid = dict(learn_rate=learn_rate, dropout_rate=dropout_rate)

# build and fit the GridSearchCV
grid = GridSearchCV(estimator = model, param_grid = param_grid, cv
= KFold(random_state=seed), verbose = 10)
grid_results = grid.fit(X_standardized, Y)

# summarize the results
print("Best: {0}, using {1}".format(grid_results.best_score_,
grid_results.best_params_))
means = grid_results.cv_results_['mean_test_score']
stds = grid_results.cv_results_['std_test_score']
params = grid_results.cv_results_['params']
for mean, stdev, param in zip(means, stds, params):
    print('{0} ({1}) with: {2}'.format(mean, stdev, param))
```

Let's now go ahead and run the cell we just created. We will see the grid search running for each of the learn rates and dropout rates that we specified. We will get the following output:

```
Fitting 3 folds for each of 9 candidates, totalling 27 fits        [CV]  dropout_rate=0.1, learn_rate=0.001, score=0.725190845154624, total=    5.7s
[CV] dropout_rate=0.0, learn_rate=0.001 .............................    [CV] dropout_rate=0.1, learn_rate=0.001 ..............................
[CV]  dropout_rate=0.0, learn_rate=0.001, score=0.748091161397337, total=  26.3s    [CV]  dropout_rate=0.1, learn_rate=0.001, score=0.763358790008864, total=    5.7s
[CV] dropout_rate=0.0, learn_rate=0.001 .............................    [CV] dropout_rate=0.1, learn_rate=0.001 ..............................

[Parallel(n_jobs=1)]: Done  1 out of  1 | elapsed:  26.4s remaining:    0.0s    [CV]  dropout_rate=0.1, learn_rate=0.001, score=0.838461536627549 4, total=    5.9s
                                                                   [CV] dropout_rate=0.1, learn_rate=0.01 ..............................
[CV]  dropout_rate=0.0, learn_rate=0.001, score=0.778625960113438, total=   5.1s    [CV]  dropout_rate=0.1, learn_rate=0.01, score=0.7404580234571267, total=    6.4s
[CV] dropout_rate=0.0, learn_rate=0.001 .............................    [CV] dropout_rate=0.1, learn_rate=0.01 ..............................

[Parallel(n_jobs=1)]: Done  2 out of  2 | elapsed:  31.6s remaining:    0.0s    [CV]  dropout_rate=0.1, learn_rate=0.01, score=0.7480916048734243, total=    6.0s
                                                                   [CV] dropout_rate=0.1, learn_rate=0.01 ..............................
[CV]  dropout_rate=0.0, learn_rate=0.001, score=0.8461538553237915, total=   5.0s    [CV]  dropout_rate=0.1, learn_rate=0.01, score=0.820769236271198, total=    6.5s
[CV] dropout_rate=0.0, learn_rate=0.01 .............................    [CV] dropout_rate=0.1, learn_rate=0.1 ..............................

[Parallel(n_jobs=1)]: Done  3 out of  3 | elapsed:  36.7s remaining:    0.0s    [CV]  dropout_rate=0.1, learn_rate=0.1, score=0.7099236600271618, total=    6.4s
                                                                   [CV] dropout_rate=0.1, learn_rate=0.1 ..............................
[CV]  dropout_rate=0.0, learn_rate=0.01, score=0.740458014357181, total=   5.0s    [CV]  dropout_rate=0.1, learn_rate=0.1, score=0.7709923736921703, total=    6.1s
[CV] dropout_rate=0.0, learn_rate=0.01 .............................    [CV] dropout_rate=0.1, learn_rate=0.1 ..............................

[Parallel(n_jobs=1)]: Done  4 out of  4 | elapsed:  41.8s remaining:    0.0s    [CV]  dropout_rate=0.1, learn_rate=0.1, score=0.7769230833420386, total=    7.1s
                                                                   [CV] dropout_rate=0.2, learn_rate=0.001 ..............................
[CV]  dropout_rate=0.0, learn_rate=0.01, score=0.7862595406197409, total=   5.0s    [CV]  dropout_rate=0.2, learn_rate=0.001, score=0.7404580152671756, total=    7.5s
[CV] dropout_rate=0.0, learn_rate=0.01 .............................    [CV] dropout_rate=0.2, learn_rate=0.001 ..............................

[Parallel(n_jobs=1)]: Done  5 out of  5 | elapsed:  46.9s remaining:    0.0s    [CV]  dropout_rate=0.2, learn_rate=0.001, score=0.7709923705071894, total=    7.3s
                                                                   [CV] dropout_rate=0.2, learn_rate=0.001 ..............................
[CV]  dropout_rate=0.0, learn_rate=0.01, score=0.7769230741720933, total=   5.1s    [CV]  dropout_rate=0.2, learn_rate=0.001, score=0.8384615457974948, total=    7.2s
[CV] dropout_rate=0.0, learn_rate=0.1 .............................    [CV] dropout_rate=0.2, learn_rate=0.01 ..............................

[Parallel(n_jobs=1)]: Done  6 out of  6 | elapsed:  52.1s remaining:    0.0s    [CV]  dropout_rate=0.2, learn_rate=0.01, score=0.740458014357181, total=    7.3s
                                                                   [CV] dropout_rate=0.2, learn_rate=0.01 ..............................
[CV]  dropout_rate=0.0, learn_rate=0.1, score=0.6946564858196346, total=   5.0s    [CV]  dropout_rate=0.2, learn_rate=0.01, score=0.770992360497249, total=    6.6s
[CV] dropout_rate=0.0, learn_rate=0.1 .............................    [CV] dropout_rate=0.2, learn_rate=0.01 ..............................

[Parallel(n_jobs=1)]: Done  7 out of  7 | elapsed:  57.2s remaining:    0.0s    [CV]  dropout_rate=0.2, learn_rate=0.01, score=0.8153846218035772, total=    6.7s
                                                                   [CV] dropout_rate=0.2, learn_rate=0.1 ..............................
[CV]  dropout_rate=0.0, learn_rate=0.1, score=0.763358779990946, total=   5.1s    [CV]  dropout_rate=0.2, learn_rate=0.1, score=0.7099236600271618, total=    6.9s
[CV] dropout_rate=0.0, learn_rate=0.1 .............................    [CV] dropout_rate=0.2, learn_rate=0.1 ..............................

[Parallel(n_jobs=1)]: Done  8 out of  8 | elapsed:  1.0min remaining:    0.0s    [CV]  dropout_rate=0.2, learn_rate=0.1, score=0.748091610788309, total=    6.8s
                                                                   [CV] dropout_rate=0.2, learn_rate=0.1 ..............................
[CV]  dropout_rate=0.0, learn_rate=0.1, score=0.800000011920929, total=   5.7s    [CV]  dropout_rate=0.2, learn_rate=0.1, score=0.699999988079071, total=    6.9s
[CV] dropout_rate=0.1, learn_rate=0.001 .............................

[Parallel(n_jobs=1)]: Done  9 out of  9 | elapsed:  1.1min remaining:    0.0s    [Parallel(n_jobs=1)]: Done  27 out of  27 | elapsed:  3.2min finished

                Best: 0.7908163351976142, using {'dropout_rate': 0.0, 'learn_rate': 0.001}
                0.7908163351976142 (0.04092945245626919) with: {'dropout_rate': 0.0, 'learn_rate': 0.001}
                0.767857411845635 (0.019701398964752953) with: {'dropout_rate': 0.0, 'learn_rate': 0.01}
                0.7525510239053745 (0.0436552908563337) with: {'dropout_rate': 0.0, 'learn_rate': 0.1}
                0.7755102090993706 (0.04700773782551412) with: {'dropout_rate': 0.1, 'learn_rate': 0.001}
                0.77295918884326 (0.04084093245867084 4) with: {'dropout_rate': 0.1, 'learn_rate': 0.01}
                0.7525510236012692 (0.03029656314273123) with: {'dropout_rate': 0.1, 'learn_rate': 0.1}
                0.78316326910 7439 (0.0409031279769419) with: {'dropout_rate': 0.2, 'learn_rate': 0.001}
                0.77551020392958 (0.030736028865651223) with: {'dropout_rate': 0.2, 'learn_rate': 0.01}
                0.7193877523650929 (0.02073466068352178) with: {'dropout_rate': 0.2, 'learn_rate': 0.1}
```

As we can see, we achieved our best outcome with a learn rate of 0.001 and no dropout regularization at all. Lowering the learning rate by just a decimal point prevented our network from overgeneralizing or overfitting too much, in a similar way to the dropout process.

Finding the optimal hyperparameters

We're now going to optimize the weight initialization that we're applying to the end of each of these neurons:

1. To do this, we will first copy the code from the cell that we ran in the previous *Reducing overfitting using dropout regularization* section, and paste it into a new one. In this section, we won't be changing the general structure of the code; instead, we will be modifying some parameters and optimizing the search.

2. We now know the best `learn_rate` and `dropout_rate`, so we are going to hardcode these and remove them. We are also going to remove the `Dropout` layers that we added in the previous section. We will modify the learning rate of the `Adam` optimizer to `0.001`, as this is the best value that we found.

3. Since we are trying to optimize the `activation` and `init` variables, we will define them in the `create_model()` function. We will also replace the `kernel_initializer` and `activation` parameters in the layers with the variables that we just defined. Our cell will now look as follows:

```
In [20]:  # Do a grid search for learning rate and dropout rate
          # import necessary packages

          # Define a random seed
          seed = 6
          np.random.seed(seed)

          # Start defining the model
          def create_model(activation, init):
              # create model
              model = Sequential()
              model.add(Dense(8, input_dim = 8, kernel_initializer= init, activation= activation))
              model.add(Dense(4, input_dim = 8, kernel_initializer= init, activation= activation))
              model.add(Dense(1, activation='sigmoid'))

              # compile the model
              adam = Adam(lr = 0.001)
              model.compile(loss = 'binary_crossentropy', optimizer = adam, metrics = ['accuracy'])
              return model

          # create the model
          model = KerasClassifier(build_fn = create_model, epochs = 100, batch_size = 20, verbose = 0)

          # define the grid search parameters
          learn_rate = [0.001, 0.01, 0.1]
          dropout_rate = [0.0, 0.1, 0.2]

          # make a dictionary of the grid search parameters
          param_grid = dict(learn_rate=learn_rate, dropout_rate=dropout_rate)

          # build and fit the GridSearchCV
          grid = GridSearchCV(estimator = model, param_grid = param_grid, cv = KFold(random_state=seed), verbose = 10)
          grid_results = grid.fit(X_standardized, Y)
```

4. We now need to define the grid search parameters for this section. We will define four activation parameters: softmax, relu, tanh, and linear. We also define three initialization parameters: uniform, normal, and zero. These will be defined as follows:

```
# define the grid search parameters
activation = ['softmax', 'relu', 'tanh', 'linear']
init = ['uniform', 'normal', 'zero']
```

We will pass these to our create_model() function.

5. Let's build our parameter grid using the dict() function, as shown in the following code block:

```
param_grid = dict(activation = activation, init = init)
```

6. It's now time to run the grid search. First, let's recap our code so far:

```
# Do a grid search to optimize kernel initialization and activation
functions

# Define a random seed
seed = 6
np.random.seed(seed)

# Start defining the model
def create_model(activation, init):   # defined variables here
    # create model
    model = Sequential()
    model.add(Dense(8, input_dim = 8, kernel_initializer= init,
activation= activation))
    model.add(Dense(4, input_dim = 8, kernel_initializer= init,
activation= activation))
    model.add(Dense(1, activation='sigmoid'))
    # compile the model
    adam = Adam(lr = 0.001)    # hardcoded the learning rate
    model.compile(loss = 'binary_crossentropy', optimizer = adam,
metrics = ['accuracy'])
    return model

# create the model
model = KerasClassifier(build_fn = create_model, epochs = 100,
batch_size = 20, verbose = 0)

# defined the grid search parameters here
activation = ['softmax', 'relu', 'tanh', 'linear']
init = ['uniform', 'normal', 'zero']
```

```
# made a dictionary of the grid search parameters here
param_grid = dict(activation = activation, init = init)

# build and fit the GridSearchCV
grid = GridSearchCV(estimator = model, param_grid = param_grid, cv
= KFold(random_state=seed), verbose = 10)
grid_results = grid.fit(X_standardized, Y)

# summarize the results
print("Best: {0}, using {1}".format(grid_results.best_score_,
grid_results.best_params_))
means = grid_results.cv_results_['mean_test_score']
stds = grid_results.cv_results_['std_test_score']
params = grid_results.cv_results_['params']
for mean, stdev, param in zip(means, stds, params):
    print('{0} ({1}) with: {2}'.format(mean, stdev, param))
```

Run the cell and find out which activation and initialization functions are optimal for our grid search. We will get the following output:

```
Fitting 3 folds for each of 12 candidates, totalling 36 fits
[CV] activation=softmax, init=uniform ......................................
[CV]  activation=softmax, init=uniform, score=0.7557252035796187, total=   5.2s
[CV] activation=softmax, init=uniform ......................................

[Parallel(n_jobs=1)]: Done   1 out of   1 | elapsed:    5.2s remaining:    0.0s

[CV]  activation=softmax, init=uniform, score=0.7557252003946378, total=   5.5s
[CV] activation=softmax, init=uniform ......................................

[Parallel(n_jobs=1)]: Done   2 out of   2 | elapsed:   10.9s remaining:    0.0s

[CV]  activation=softmax, init=uniform, score=0.8153846218035772, total=   6.5s
[CV] activation=softmax, init=normal ......................................

[Parallel(n_jobs=1)]: Done   3 out of   3 | elapsed:   17.4s remaining:    0.0s

[CV]  activation=softmax, init=normal, score=0.6106870242657553, total=   6.1s
[CV] activation=softmax, init=normal ......................................

[Parallel(n_jobs=1)]: Done   4 out of   4 | elapsed:   23.6s remaining:    0.0s

[CV]  activation=softmax, init=normal, score=0.7557252003946378, total=   5.7s
[CV] activation=softmax, init=normal ......................................

[Parallel(n_jobs=1)]: Done   5 out of   5 | elapsed:   29.4s remaining:    0.0s

[CV]  activation=softmax, init=normal, score=0.8230769267449012, total=   5.1s
[CV] activation=softmax, init=zero ......................................

[Parallel(n_jobs=1)]: Done   6 out of   6 | elapsed:   34.6s remaining:    0.0s

[CV]  activation=softmax, init=zero, score=0.6106870242657553, total=   5.2s
[CV] activation=softmax, init=zero ......................................

[Parallel(n_jobs=1)]: Done   7 out of   7 | elapsed:   40.0s remaining:    0.0s

[CV]  activation=softmax, init=zero, score=0.6948584958295749, total=   5.5s
[CV] activation=softmax, init=zero ......................................

[Parallel(n_jobs=1)]: Done   8 out of   8 | elapsed:   45.5s remaining:    0.0s

[CV] activation=relu, init=uniform ......................................

[Parallel(n_jobs=1)]: Done   9 out of   9 | elapsed:   50.8s remaining:    0.0s

[CV]  activation=relu, init=uniform, score=0.7328244347608727, total=   5.5s
[CV] activation=relu, init=uniform ......................................
[CV]  activation=relu, init=uniform, score=0.7480916107883389, total=   5.3s
[CV] activation=relu, init=uniform ......................................
[CV]  activation=relu, init=uniform, score=0.8230769221599286, total=   5.6s
[CV] activation=relu, init=normal ......................................
[CV]  activation=relu, init=normal, score=0.725190351448836, total=   5.4s
[CV] activation=relu, init=normal ......................................
[CV]  activation=relu, init=normal, score=0.7709923705071894, total=   5.5s
[CV] activation=relu, init=normal ......................................
[CV]  activation=relu, init=normal, score=0.8461538599087641, total=   5.6s
[CV] activation=relu, init=zero ......................................
[CV]  activation=relu, init=zero, score=0.6106870242657553, total=   5.7s
[CV] activation=relu, init=zero ......................................
[CV]  activation=relu, init=zero, score=0.6948584958295749, total=   5.8s
[CV] activation=relu, init=zero ......................................
[CV]  activation=relu, init=zero, score=0.699999988079071, total=   5.9s
[CV] activation=tanh, init=uniform ......................................
[CV]  activation=tanh, init=uniform, score=0.7557251944479673, total=   6.3s
[CV] activation=tanh, init=uniform ......................................
[CV]  activation=tanh, init=uniform, score=0.7709923796071351, total=   6.1s
[CV] activation=tanh, init=uniform ......................................
[CV]  activation=tanh, init=uniform, score=0.8230769267449012, total=   6.4s
[CV] activation=tanh, init=normal ......................................
[CV]  activation=tanh, init=normal, score=0.7633587840859218, total=   6.1s
[CV] activation=tanh, init=normal ......................................
[CV]  activation=tanh, init=normal, score=0.7786259692133838, total=   6.4s
[CV] activation=tanh, init=normal ......................................
[CV]  activation=tanh, init=normal, score=0.838461536627549494, total=   7.1s
[CV] activation=tanh, init=zero ......................................
[CV]  activation=tanh, init=zero, score=0.6106870242657553, total=   7.3s
[CV] activation=tanh, init=zero ......................................
[CV]  activation=tanh, init=zero, score=0.6948584958295749, total=   6.9s
[CV] activation=tanh, init=zero ......................................
[CV]  activation=tanh, init=zero, score=0.699999988079071, total=   6.8s
[CV] activation=linear, init=uniform ......................................
[CV]  activation=linear, init=uniform, score=0.7709923645922245, total=   7.1s
[CV] activation=linear, init=uniform ......................................
[CV]  activation=linear, init=uniform, score=0.7633587900008864, total=   6.8s
[CV] activation=linear, init=uniform ......................................
[CV]  activation=linear, init=uniform, score=0.8461538553237915, total=   7.0s
[CV] activation=linear, init=normal ......................................
[CV]  activation=linear, init=normal, score=0.7709923554922788, total=   7.3s
[CV] activation=linear, init=normal ......................................
[CV]  activation=linear, init=normal, score=0.7633587900008864, total=   7.2s
[CV] activation=linear, init=normal ......................................
[CV]  activation=linear, init=normal, score=0.8384615457974948, total=   7.5s
[CV] activation=linear, init=zero ......................................
[CV]  activation=linear, init=zero, score=0.6106870242657553, total=   7.3s
[CV] activation=linear, init=zero ......................................
[CV]  activation=linear, init=zero, score=0.6948584958295749, total=   7.5s
[CV] activation=linear, init=zero ......................................
[CV]  activation=linear, init=zero, score=0.699999988079071, total=   7.6s

[Parallel(n_jobs=1)]: Done  36 out of  36 | elapsed:  3.8min finished

Best: 0.7933673531729348, using {'activation': 'tanh', 'init': 'normal'}
0.7755102136609505 (0.026087641954935023) with: {'activation': 'softmax', 'init': 'uniform'}
0.7295918416003792 (0.08860775018104312) with: {'activation': 'softmax', 'init': 'normal'}
0.6668367345874468 (0.040922317011154695) with: {'activation': 'softmax', 'init': 'zero'}
0.7678571475707755 (0.03939442059435707) with: {'activation': 'relu', 'init': 'uniform'}
0.7806122493074865 (0.04981944702508574) with: {'activation': 'relu', 'init': 'normal'}
0.6668367345874468 (0.040922317011154695) with: {'activation': 'relu', 'init': 'zero'}
0.7831632721484924 (0.0287995885934298) with: {'activation': 'tanh', 'init': 'uniform'}
0.7933673531729348 (0.032371719468448684) with: {'activation': 'tanh', 'init': 'normal'}
0.6668367345874468 (0.040922317011154695) with: {'activation': 'tanh', 'init': 'zero'}
0.7933673531729348 (0.037313655933021314) with: {'activation': 'linear', 'init': 'uniform'}
0.7908163291155076 (0.03370016593390863) with: {'activation': 'linear', 'init': 'normal'}
0.6668367345874468 (0.040922317011154695) with: {'activation': 'linear', 'init': 'zero'}
```

From the preceding screenshot, we find that the `tanh` activation function performs the best when coupled with a `normal` initialization function. We can now use these to our advantage in order to fine-tune the neurons in the following section.

Optimizing the number of neurons

Let's now move on to tuning the number of neurons in each of these layers. Since we are following the same steps as the preceding sections, we will go through all these steps and do a recap with the code snippet at the end. So, let's get started with the following steps:

1. We will start by copying the code from the cell used in the *Finding the optimal hyperparameters* section, and paste it in a new cell. In this new cell, we will play around with the number of neurons by modifying some of the variables.

2. We will convert the total number of neurons present in each hidden layer into variables, such as `neuron1` and `neuron2`. We will also define these variables in the `create_model()` function, so that they are called every time we execute it.

3. We will also change the `kernel_initializer` and `activation` values to `tanh` and `normal`, since those were the ones that performed best, as we saw in the *Finding the optimal hyperparameters* section.

4. We will define the grid search parameters as `4,8,16` for `neuron1`, and `2,4,8` for `neuron2`.

5. Our next step is to create a dictionary of the parameters using the following code snippet:

```
param_grid = dict(neuron1 = neuron1, neuron2 = neuron2)
```

6. One final step, before we train the model, is to add the following command in the `GridSearchCV()` function:

```
refit = True
```

This tells the system to retrain the model with the best parameters that we find.

7. Let's recap our code:

```
# Do a grid search to find the optimal number of neurons in each
hidden layer
# Define a random seed
seed = 6
np.random.seed(seed)

# Start defining the model
```

```
def create_model(neuron1, neuron2):
    # create model
    model = Sequential()
    model.add(Dense(neuron1, input_dim = 8, kernel_initializer=
'uniform', activation= 'linear'))
    model.add(Dense(neuron2, input_dim = neuron1,
kernel_initializer= 'uniform', activation= 'linear'))
    model.add(Dense(1, activation='sigmoid'))
    # compile the model
    adam = Adam(lr = 0.001)
    model.compile(loss = 'binary_crossentropy', optimizer = adam,
metrics = ['accuracy'])
    return model

# create the model
model = KerasClassifier(build_fn = create_model, epochs = 100,
batch_size = 20, verbose = 0)

# define the grid search parameters
neuron1 = [4, 8, 16]
neuron2 = [2, 4, 8]

# make a dictionary of the grid search parameters
param_grid = dict(neuron1 = neuron1, neuron2 = neuron2)

# build and fit the GridSearchCV
grid = GridSearchCV(estimator = model, param_grid = param_grid, cv
= KFold(random_state=seed), refit = True, verbose = 10)
grid_results = grid.fit(X_standardized, Y)

# summarize the results
print("Best: {0}, using {1}".format(grid_results.best_score_,
grid_results.best_params_))
means = grid_results.cv_results_['mean_test_score']
stds = grid_results.cv_results_['std_test_score']
params = grid_results.cv_results_['params']
for mean, stdev, param in zip(means, stds, params):
    print('{0} ({1}) with: {2}'.format(mean, stdev, param))
```

8. We will now run this cell. This results in the following output:

```
Fitting 3 folds for each of 9 candidates, totalling 27 fits
[CV] neuron1=4, neuron2=2 ......................................
[CV] ... neuron1=4, neuron2=2, score=0.7709923645922245, total=  14.9s
[CV] neuron1=4, neuron2=2 ......................................

[Parallel(n_jobs=1)]: Done   1 out of   1 | elapsed:   15.0s remaining:   0.0s

[CV] ... neuron1=4, neuron2=2, score=0.7633587900008864, total=  13.3s
[CV] neuron1=4, neuron2=2 ......................................

[Parallel(n_jobs=1)]: Done   2 out of   2 | elapsed:   28.4s remaining:   0.0s

[CV] ... neuron1=4, neuron2=2, score=0.8230769267449012, total=  17.4s
[CV] neuron1=4, neuron2=4 ......................................

[Parallel(n_jobs=1)]: Done   3 out of   3 | elapsed:   46.0s remaining:   0.0s

[CV] ... neuron1=4, neuron2=4, score=0.7709923645922245, total=  11.5s
[CV] neuron1=4, neuron2=4 ......................................

[Parallel(n_jobs=1)]: Done   4 out of   4 | elapsed:   57.6s remaining:   0.0s

[CV] ... neuron1=4, neuron2=4, score=0.7786259692133838, total=  10.7s
[CV] neuron1=4, neuron2=4 ......................................

[Parallel(n_jobs=1)]: Done   5 out of   5 | elapsed:  1.1min remaining:   0.0s

[CV] ... neuron1=4, neuron2=4, score=0.8153846218035772, total=  11.3s
[CV] neuron1=4, neuron2=8 ......................................

[Parallel(n_jobs=1)]: Done   6 out of   6 | elapsed:  1.3min remaining:   0.0s

[CV] ... neuron1=4, neuron2=8, score=0.7633587749859759, total=  17.1s
[CV] neuron1=4, neuron2=8 ......................................

[Parallel(n_jobs=1)]: Done   7 out of   7 | elapsed:  1.6min remaining:   0.0s

[CV] ... neuron1=4, neuron2=8, score=0.7633587900008864, total=  13.7s
[CV] neuron1=4, neuron2=8 ......................................

[Parallel(n_jobs=1)]: Done   8 out of   8 | elapsed:  1.8min remaining:   0.0s

[CV] .... neuron1=4, neuron2=8, score=0.830769236271198, total=  12.5s
[CV] neuron1=8, neuron2=2 ......................................

[Parallel(n_jobs=1)]: Done   9 out of   9 | elapsed:  2.1min remaining:   0.0s

[CV] ... neuron1=8, neuron2=2, score=0.7633587840859216, total=  17.1s
[CV] neuron1=8, neuron2=2 ......................................
```

```
[CV] ... neuron1=8, neuron2=2, score=0.7633587900008864, total=  13.9s
[CV] neuron1=8, neuron2=2 ......................................
[CV] ... neuron1=8, neuron2=2, score=0.8384615457974948, total=  18.5s
[CV] neuron1=8, neuron2=4 ......................................
[CV] ... neuron1=8, neuron2=4, score=0.7633587749859759, total=  17.8s
[CV] neuron1=8, neuron2=4 ......................................
[CV] ... neuron1=8, neuron2=4, score=0.7633587900008864, total=  14.4s
[CV] neuron1=8, neuron2=4 ......................................
[CV] ... neuron1=8, neuron2=4, score=0.8384615457974948, total=  12.0s
[CV] neuron1=8, neuron2=8 ......................................
[CV] ... neuron1=8, neuron2=8, score=0.7633587840859216, total=  11.5s
[CV] neuron1=8, neuron2=8 ......................................
[CV] ... neuron1=8, neuron2=8, score=0.7633587900008864, total=  11.7s
[CV] neuron1=8, neuron2=8 ......................................
[CV] .... neuron1=8, neuron2=8, score=0.830769236271198, total=  12.3s
[CV] neuron1=16, neuron2=2 .....................................
[CV] .. neuron1=16, neuron2=2, score=0.7633587840859216, total=  13.5s
[CV] neuron1=16, neuron2=2 .....................................
[CV] .. neuron1=16, neuron2=2, score=0.7633587900008864, total=  14.7s
[CV] neuron1=16, neuron2=2 .....................................
[CV] .. neuron1=16, neuron2=2, score=0.8461538553237915, total=  13.2s
[CV] neuron1=16, neuron2=4 .....................................
[CV] .. neuron1=16, neuron2=4, score=0.7709923645922245, total=  12.7s
[CV] neuron1=16, neuron2=4 .....................................
[CV] .. neuron1=16, neuron2=4, score=0.7633587900008864, total=  13.9s
[CV] neuron1=16, neuron2=4 .....................................
[CV] ... neuron1=16, neuron2=4, score=0.838461541212522, total=  12.4s
[CV] neuron1=16, neuron2=8 .....................................
[CV] .. neuron1=16, neuron2=8, score=0.7633587840859216, total=  12.7s
[CV] neuron1=16, neuron2=8 .....................................
[CV] .. neuron1=16, neuron2=8, score=0.7633587900008864, total=  12.3s
[CV] neuron1=16, neuron2=8 .....................................
[CV] ... neuron1=16, neuron2=8, score=0.830769236271198, total=  2.9min

[Parallel(n_jobs=1)]: Done  27 out of  27 | elapsed: 8.9min finished

Best: 0.7908163351976142, using {'neuron1': 16, 'neuron2': 2}
0.785714290123813 (0.02650267677503863) with: {'neuron1': 4, 'neuron2': 2}
0.7882653126607135 (0.019356087898682556) with: {'neuron1': 4, 'neuron2': 4}
0.785714290123813 (0.03173682706663349) with: {'neuron1': 4, 'neuron2': 8}
0.7882653141812402 (0.03535836258886925) with: {'neuron1': 8, 'neuron2': 2}
0.7882653111401869 (0.03535836473101593) with: {'neuron1': 8, 'neuron2': 4}
0.7857142931648663 (0.031736824926506764) with: {'neuron1': 8, 'neuron2': 8}
0.7908163351976142 (0.03897990025127174) with: {'neuron1': 16, 'neuron2': 2}
0.7908163306360342 (0.03370616199600475) with: {'neuron1': 16, 'neuron2': 4}
0.7857142931648663 (0.031736824926506764) with: {'neuron1': 16, 'neuron2': 8}
```

In the preceding screenshot, we find that having 16 and 2 neurons is best. We retrained our algorithm, using 16 neurons in the first layer and 2 in the second.

Generating predictions using optimal hyperparameters

We know now some optimal hyperparameters for our grid search. We will use these to predict the onset of diabetes for the patients in our dataset. To do this, we will carry out the following steps:

1. We will predict whether diabetes will occur for every example in the dataset by using the predict() function, as shown in the following code snippet:

```
# generate predictions with optimal hyperparameters
y_pred = grid.predict(X_standardized)
```

2. We will then use the `.shape` command to see what the predictions look like. The following screenshot shows the output for this step:

```
In [23]:  print(y_pred.shape)

          (392, 1)
```

From the preceding screenshot, we can see that there are `392` predictions with a numerical value for each.

3. Let's print off the first five and see what they look like. We get the following output:

```
In [24]:  print(y_pred[:5])

          [[0]
           [1]
           [0]
           [1]
           [1]]
```

4. We are now going to do a classification report and get an accuracy score for the predictions, so that we can better understand our results. This can be done as follows:

```
from sklearn.metrics import classification_report, accuracy_score
print(accuracy_score(Y, y_pred))
print(classification_report(Y, y_pred))
```

We will get the following output:

```
In [25]:  # Generate a classification report
          from sklearn.metrics import classification_report, accuracy_score

          print(accuracy_score(Y, y_pred))
          print(classification_report(Y, y_pred))

          0.7806122448979592
                        precision    recall  f1-score   support

                     0       0.81      0.89      0.84       262
                     1       0.71      0.57      0.63       130

          avg / total       0.77      0.78      0.77       392
```

From the preceding output, we can see that we were able to predict whether patients would have diabetes correctly 78% of the time. The **precision** refers to the classifier's ability to label a negative sample correctly as negative, instead of as a false positive. Since precision for the negative samples is 71%, we do have some false positives, which is unfortunate.

Similarly, **recall** refers to the classifier's ability to find the positive samples. This also accounts for false negatives. We actually had a lot of false negatives here, which might be a good thing: we don't necessarily want to tell a healthy individual that they have diabetes incorrectly. At the same time, however, we're missing a lot of the people who do have diabetes.

Support refers to the number of instances for each class. We find that 0 was predicted 262 times, which means that 262 individuals were predicted as healthy. We had 130 individuals who were predicted to have diabetes.

Bonus step

Let's take a look at an example to predict whether or not a patient has diabetes:

1. To do this, we will first run the following code snippet:

```
example = df.iloc[1]
print(example)
```

This gives us a DataFrame for a patient with `1` as the `class` label, shown in the following screenshot:

```
In [23]:  example = df.iloc[1]
          print(example)

          n_pregnant                        0.000
          glucose_concentration           137.000
          blood_pressure (mm Hg)           40.000
          skin_thickness (mm)              35.000
          serum_insulin (mu U/ml)         168.000
          BMI                              43.100
          pedigree_function                 2.288
          age                              33.000
          class                             1.000
          Name: 4, dtype: float64
```

2. Now, we're going to make a prediction using our optimized deep neural network. To do that, we will run the following code snippet:

```
prediction = grid.predict(X_standardized[1].reshape(1, -1))
print(prediction)
```

This gives us the following output:

```
In [27]:  prediction = grid.predict(X_standardized[1].reshape(1, -1))
          print(prediction)

          [[1]]
```

As seen in the output, we have predicted correctly that this individual is likely to have diabetes.

Summary

In this chapter, we built a deep neural network in Keras and we found the optimal hyperparameters using the scikit-learn grid search. We also learned how to optimize a network by tuning the hyperparameters. Note that the results that we get might not be the same for all of us, but as long as we get similar predictions, we can consider our model a success. When you start training on new data, or if you're trying to address a different problem with a different dataset, you will have to go through this process again. In this chapter, we also learned about deep learning and hyperparameter optimization and explored how to apply them to the network to predict the onset of diabetes on a huge dataset of patients.

In the next chapter, we will look at how to classify DNA using machine algorithms.

3
DNA Classification

In this chapter, we will explore the world of bioinformatics. We will use Markov models, k-nearest neighbors algorithms, support vector machines, and other common classifiers, to classify short E. coli DNA sequences. For this project, will use a dataset from the UCI machine learning repository that has 106 DNA sequences, with 57 sequential nucleotides each. You will learn how to import data from the UCI repository, convert text input to numerical data, build and train classification algorithms, and compare and contrast classification machine learning algorithms.

We will cover the following topics:

- Classifying DNA sequences
- Data preprocessing

Classifying DNA sequences

Let's classify DNA sequences by performing the following steps:

1. Let's start a new Python Jupyter Notebook and name it DNA Classification. As always, one of the first steps that we want to take is to import the libraries and the modules that we need, and check the versions, in order to make sure that we're on the same page and that we don't make any errors while importing the modules. If we do, we can go back and install them again.

   Take a look at the following code snippet:

   ```
   import sys
   import numpy
   import sklearn
   import pandas

   print('Python: {}'.format(sys.version))
   print('Numpy: {}'.format(numpy.__version__))
   ```

```
print('Sklearn: {}'.format(sklearn.__version__))
print('Pandas: {}'.format(pandas.__version__))
```

The preceding code snippet will import all of the necessary libraries, and will indicate which versions we are using as shown in the following screenshot:

```
Python: 3.6.5 |Anaconda, Inc.| (default, Mar 29 2018, 13:32:41) [MSC v.1900 64 bit (AMD64)]
Numpy: 1.14.3
Sklearn: 0.19.1
Pandas: 0.23.0
```

2. After that, we'll install `numpy`, `pandas`, and the UCI repository dataset that we will be using in this chapter. The dataset is the Molecular Biology (Promoter Gene Sequences) dataset, which can be found at `https://archive.ics.uci.edu/ml/machine-learning-databases/molecular-biology/promoter-gene-sequences/`.

3. Next, we will classify dataset by the class, ID, and sequence, as follows:

```
import numpy as np
import pandas as pd
url =
'https://archive.ics.uci.edu/ml/machine-learning-databases/molecula
r-biology/promoter-gene-sequences/promoters.data'
names = ['Class', 'id', 'Sequence']
data = pd.read_csv(url, names = names)
```

4. Print the first five instances using the `iloc[]` method, as shown in the following screenshot:

```
In [3]:  print(data.iloc[0])

         Class                                                              +
         id                                                              S10
         Sequence      \t\ttactagcaatacgcttgcgttcggtggttaagtatgtataat...
         Name: 0, dtype: object
```

In the preceding screenshot of output, we can see \t\ at the start of every sequence. That is because there's a tab or two preceding every sequence in the CSV file, and they are being recorded as we import the data.

Data preprocessing

We will build our dataset using a custom `pandas` DataFrame and then we will redefine the DataFrame based on the information that we have imported. Each column in a DataFrame is called a **series**. We will start by making a series for each column, using the `data.loc[]` method, and then printing the first five classes as shown in the following code snippet:

```
classes = data.loc[:, 'Class']
print(classes[:5])
```

In the first five rows, we have the `Class` column, all pluses (+) or minuses (-). The pluses, in this case, are the promoters, while the minuses are anything that isn't a promoter. Take a look at the following screenshot:

```
0      +
1      +
2      +
3      +
4      +
Name: Class, dtype: object
```

Generating a DNA sequence

Let's generate a DNA sequence by executing the following steps:

1. Now we will generate a list of DNA sequences, loop through the sequences, and split them into individual nucleotides, because we want these to be the input for our algorithm.

2. We remove the tab characters, append the class assignment, and add the nucleotides to the dataset, as follows:

```
sequences = list(data.loc[:, 'Sequence'])
dataset = {}
for i, seq in enumerate(sequences):
nucleotides = list(seq)
nucleotides = [x for x in nucleotides if x != '\t']
nucleotides.append(classes[i])
dataset[i] = nucleotides
print(dataset[0])
```

We now have all of our different columns. Each column contains either an individual nucleotide or a base pair. The nucleotides are thymine (t), adenine (a), cytosine (c), and guanine (g). We also have the appended class at the end, which is denoted by the + as shown in the following screenshot:

```
['t', 'a', 'c', 't', 'a', 'g', 'c', 'a', 'a', 't', 'a', 'c', 'g', 'c', 't', 't', 'g', 'c',
 'g', 't', 't', 'c', 'g', 'g', 't', 'g', 'g', 't', 't', 'a', 'a', 'g', 't', 'a', 't', 'g',
 't', 'a', 't', 'a', 'a', 't', 'g', 'c', 'g', 'c', 'g', 'g', 'g', 'c', 't', 't', 'g', 't',
 'c', 'g', 't', '+']
```

3. Let's turn this data back into `DataFrame` and print it, to see what it looks like:

```
dframe = pd.DataFrame(dataset)
print(dframe)
```

As you can see in the following screenshot, we have 106 columns (which are the individual nucleotides), and 58 rows:

	0	1	2	3	4	5	6	7	8	9	...	96	97	98	99	100	101	102	103	104	105
0	t	t	g	a	t	a	c	t	c	t	...	c	c	t	a	g	c	g	c	c	t
1	a	g	t	a	c	g	a	t	g	t	...	c	g	a	g	a	c	t	g	t	a
2	c	c	a	t	g	g	g	t	a	t	...	g	c	t	a	g	t	a	c	c	a
3	t	t	c	t	a	g	g	c	c	t	...	a	t	g	g	a	c	t	g	g	c
4	a	a	t	g	t	g	g	t	t	a	...	g	a	a	g	g	a	t	a	t	a
5	g	t	a	t	a	c	g	a	t	a	...	t	g	c	g	c	a	c	c	c	t
6	c	c	g	g	a	a	g	c	a	a	...	a	g	c	t	a	t	t	t	c	t
7	a	c	a	a	t	a	t	a	a	t	...	g	a	g	g	t	g	c	a	t	a
8	a	t	g	t	t	g	g	a	t	t	...	a	c	a	t	g	g	a	c	c	a
9	t	g	a	g	a	g	g	a	a	t	...	c	t	a	a	t	c	a	g	a	t
10	a	a	a	t	a	a	a	a	t	c	...	c	t	c	c	c	c	c	a	a	a
11	c	c	c	g	c	g	g	c	a	c	...	c	t	g	t	a	t	a	t	t	a
12	g	a	t	t	t	g	g	a	c	t	...	t	c	a	c	g	c	a	g	g	a
13	c	g	a	a	a	a	a	c	t	c	...	t	t	g	c	c	t	g	a	g	t
14	t	t	g	t	t	t	t	t	g	t	...	a	t	t	a	c	a	a	g	c	a
15	t	t	t	c	t	g	t	t	c	t	...	g	g	c	a	t	a	t	a	c	a
16	g	g	g	g	g	g	t	g	g	g	...	a	t	a	g	c	a	t	t	t	g
17	c	t	c	a	a	a	a	a	a	t	...	g	t	a	a	g	c	a	g	c	g

We would actually rather have this in a different orientation.

4. Let's switch the rows and columns using the `transpose()` function and print the first five instances, as follows:

```
df = dframe.transpose()
print(df.iloc[:5])
```

We now have each instance as a row. We have 58 columns—one for each of the 57 nucleotides, and one for the class, which is either a plus or a minus as shown in the following screenshot:

	0	1	2	3	4	5	6	7	8	9	...	48	49	50	51	52	53	54	55	56	57
0	t	a	c	t	a	g	c	a	a	t	...	g	c	t	t	g	t	c	g	t	+
1	t	g	c	t	a	t	c	c	t	g	...	c	a	t	c	g	c	c	a	a	+
2	g	t	a	c	t	a	g	a	g	a	...	c	a	c	c	c	g	g	c	g	+
3	a	a	t	t	g	t	g	a	t	g	...	a	a	c	a	a	a	c	t	c	+
4	t	c	g	a	t	a	a	t	t	a	...	c	c	g	t	g	g	t	a	g	+

```
[5 rows x 58 columns]
```

5. To avoid confusion, let's rename the last column as `Class`, and print the first five instances, to see whether this worked correctly:

```
df.rename(columns = {57: 'Class'}, inplace = True)
print(df.iloc[:5])
```

We now have 57 nucleotide columns, and a final column, `Class`, shown as follows:

	0	1	2	3	4	5	6	7	8	9	...	48	49	50	51	52	53	54	55	56	Class
0	t	a	c	t	a	g	c	a	a	t	...	g	c	t	t	g	t	c	g	t	+
1	t	g	c	t	a	t	c	c	t	g	...	c	a	t	c	g	c	c	a	a	+
2	g	t	a	c	t	a	g	a	g	a	...	c	a	c	c	c	g	g	c	g	+
3	a	a	t	t	g	t	g	a	t	g	...	a	a	c	a	a	a	c	t	c	+
4	t	c	g	a	t	a	a	t	t	a	...	c	c	g	t	g	g	t	a	g	+

```
[5 rows x 58 columns]
```

6. Let's run the `df.describe()` method to learn a bit more about the data. This will give us some information about the dataset, as follows:

	0	1	2	3	4	5	6	7	8	9	...	48	49	50	51	52	53	54	55	56	Class
count	106	106	106	106	106	106	106	106	106	106	...	106	106	106	106	106	106	106	106	106	106
unique	4	4	4	4	4	4	4	4	4	4	...	4	4	4	4	4	4	4	4	4	2
top	t	a	a	c	a	a	a	a	a	a	...	c	c	c	t	t	c	c	c	t	-
freq	38	34	30	30	36	42	38	34	33	36	...	36	42	31	33	35	32	29	29	34	53

4 rows × 58 columns

From the preceding screenshot, we see the row named `top`, and we can see the letters that correspond to the different nucleotides. For each of the nucleotides, you can see that the `unique` value is 4. The `top` row shows the most common nucleotide at each position, while the `freq` row shows the amount of times that this nucleotide appeared. We have 53 promoters and 53 non-promoters in this dataset, which is a nice 50/50 split. However, we need to convert the promoter and non-promoters to numerical values. We will record the value counts for each sequence and print the details, so that we can further understand our data:

```
series = []
for name in df.columns:
  series.append(df[name].value_counts())

info = pd.DataFrame(series)
details = info.transpose()
print(details)
```

In the following screenshot, we see that the class is no longer a number; we only have pluses and minuses. We can also see the number of occurrences in each case. There aren't any pluses or minuses in the first 57 columns, which makes sense, because those should be nucleotides. We have a fairly even split in the value counts for each nucleotide in each position.

```
          0     1     2     3     4     5     6     7     8     9   ...      48   \
t      38.0  26.0  27.0  26.0  22.0  24.0  30.0  32.0  32.0  28.0  ...    21.0
c      27.0  22.0  21.0  30.0  19.0  18.0  21.0  20.0  22.0  22.0  ...    36.0
a      26.0  34.0  30.0  22.0  36.0  42.0  38.0  34.0  33.0  36.0  ...    23.0
g      15.0  24.0  28.0  28.0  29.0  22.0  17.0  20.0  19.0  20.0  ...    26.0
-       NaN   NaN   NaN   NaN   NaN   NaN   NaN   NaN   NaN   NaN  ...     NaN
+       NaN   NaN   NaN   NaN   NaN   NaN   NaN   NaN   NaN   NaN  ...     NaN

         49    50    51    52    53    54    55    56  Class
t      22.0  23.0  33.0  35.0  30.0  23.0  29.0  34.0    NaN
c      42.0  31.0  32.0  21.0  32.0  29.0  29.0  17.0    NaN
a      24.0  28.0  27.0  25.0  22.0  26.0  24.0  27.0    NaN
g      18.0  24.0  14.0  25.0  22.0  28.0  24.0  28.0    NaN
-       NaN   NaN   NaN   NaN   NaN   NaN   NaN   NaN   53.0
+       NaN   NaN   NaN   NaN   NaN   NaN   NaN   NaN   53.0

[6 rows x 58 columns]
```

We can also see that every column has either a number or a +/– label in the `Class` column. We now know that we're not missing any data, and we can move on to convert the data that we have to numerical data.

7. Let's switch to numerical data, using the `pd.get_dummies()` function. We will call the new DataFrame `numerical_df`, and we will print the first five rows:

```
numerical_df = pd.get_dummies(df)
numerical_df.iloc[:5]
```

Take a look at the following screenshot:

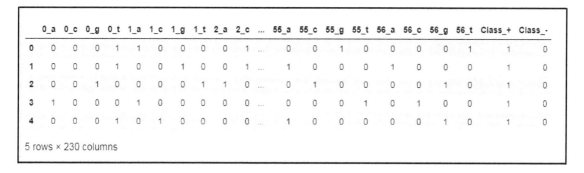

	0_a	0_c	0_g	0_t	1_a	1_c	1_g	1_t	2_a	2_c	...	55_a	55_c	55_g	55_t	56_a	56_c	56_g	56_t	Class_+	Class_-
0	0	0	0	1	1	0	0	0	0	1	...	0	0	1	0	0	0	0	1	1	0
1	0	0	0	1	0	0	1	0	0	1	...	1	0	0	0	1	0	0	0	1	0
2	0	0	1	0	0	0	0	1	1	0	...	0	1	0	0	0	0	1	0	1	0
3	1	0	0	0	1	0	0	0	0	0	...	0	0	0	1	0	1	0	0	1	0
4	0	0	0	1	0	1	0	0	0	0	...	1	0	0	0	0	0	1	0	1	0

5 rows × 230 columns

8. We are going to use an underscore to provide different text labels, to indicate the four different positions. For column 0, we have four different options: adenine, cytosine, guanine, and thymine. The 1 is placed in the relevant position of the nucleotide. In the 0 position, our first instance has thymine. In the second position, it has adenine, and so on.

Everything is binary—either a 0 or a 1—for all of the 57 positions. In each case, we have a 1 under the nucleotide that is in that particular position. This makes up a nucleotide sequence.

At the end, we have Class_+ and Class_-. This is a bit redundant; if we know that it's in the first class, we know that it's not going to be in the second.

9. Let's remove one of the Class columns and rename the remaining column to Class:

```
df = numerical_df.drop(columns=['Class_-'])
df.rename(columns = {'Class_+': 'Class'}, inplace = True)
print(df.iloc[:5])
```

Take a look at the following screenshot:

	0_a	0_c	0_g	0_t	1_a	1_c	1_g	1_t	2_a	2_c	...	54_t	55_a	55_c	\
0	0	0	0	1	1	0	0	0	0	1	...	0	0	0	
1	0	0	0	1	0	0	1	0	0	1	...	0	1	0	
2	0	0	1	0	0	0	0	1	1	0	...	0	0	1	
3	1	0	0	0	1	0	0	0	0	0	...	0	0	0	
4	0	0	0	1	0	1	0	0	0	0	...	1	1	0	

	55_g	55_t	56_a	56_c	56_g	56_t	Class
0	1	0	0	0	0	1	1
1	0	0	1	0	0	0	1
2	0	0	0	0	1	0	1
3	0	1	0	1	0	0	1
4	0	0	0	0	1	0	1

```
[5 rows x 229 columns]
```

We can now see that the last column is Class. We don't have the pluses or minuses. Now, a 1 represents a promoter class, while a 0 represents a non-promoter class.

10. Let's print location `60` and take a look at the result, as follows:

```
df = numerical_df.drop(columns=['Class_-'])

df.rename(columns = {'Class_+': 'Class'}, inplace = True)
print(df.iloc[60])
```

Take a look at the following screenshot:

0_a	0	49_t	1
0_c	0	50_a	0
0_g	1	50_c	0
0_t	0	50_g	1
1_a	1	50_t	0
1_c	0	51_a	0
1_g	0	51_c	0
1_t	0	51_g	1
2_a	0	51_t	0
2_c	0	52_a	0
2_g	1	52_c	0
2_t	0	52_g	0
3_a	0	52_t	1
3_c	0	53_a	1
3_g	1	53_c	0
3_t	0	53_g	0
4_a	0	53_t	0
4_c	0	54_a	0
4_g	0	54_c	0
4_t	1	54_g	0
5_a	0	54_t	1
5_c	0	55_a	0
5_g	1	55_c	0
5_t	0	55_g	0
6_a	0	55_t	1
6_c	0	56_a	1
6_g	1	56_c	0
6_t	0	56_g	0
7_a	0	56_t	0
7_c	1	Class	0
	..	Name: 60, Length: 229, dtype: uint8	

Thus from the preceding screenshot, we have a 0 for Class, meaning that this is a non-promoter. We now have 229 columns, 228 of which represent different nucleotide inputs (because we have four for each position). We've maintained the same information that we had before, but the dataset is now preprocessed in the way that we need it: converted to numerical input, based on the text information that was supplied from the UCI repository.

We can now move on to actually doing the machine learning, the first step of which will be to split our dataset into training and testing datasets.

Splitting the dataset

Now let's split the dataset by performing the following steps:

1. First, we need to import the algorithms from the `sklearn` library, in order to work with the dataset as follows:

```
from sklearn.neighbors import KNeighborsClassifier
from sklearn.neural_network import MLPClassifier
from sklearn.gaussian_process import GaussianProcessClassifier
from sklearn.gaussian_process.kernels import RBF
from sklearn.tree import DecisionTreeClassifier
from sklearn.ensemble import RandomForestClassifier,
AdaBoostClassifier
from sklearn.naive_bayes import GaussianNB
from sklearn.svm import SVC
from sklearn.metrics import classification_report, accurac
```

 To learn more about these algorithms, it is recommended that you take a look at the `sklearn` documentation at `http://scikit-learn.org/` `stable/documentation.html`.

2. We will now import the `model_selection` algorithm from `sklearn` and define a seed for reproducibility. After that, we'll split the data into training and testing datasets as follows:

```
from sklearn import model_selection

# Create X and Y datasets for training
X = np.array(df.drop(['Class'], 1))
y = np.array(df['Class'])

# define seed for reproducibility
seed = 1

# split data into training and testing datasets
X_train, X_test, y_train, y_test =
model_selection.train_test_split(X, y, test_size=0.25,
random_state=seed)
```

3. Next, we will define the `scoring` method and the models to train. We will evaluate each model, as follows:

```
# define scoring method
scoring = 'accuracy'

# Define models to train
names = ["Nearest Neighbors", "Gaussian Process",
         "Decision Tree", "Random Forest", "Neural Net",
"AdaBoost",
         "Naive Bayes", "SVM Linear", "SVM RBF", "SVM Sigmoid"]

classifiers = [
    KNeighborsClassifier(n_neighbors = 3),
    GaussianProcessClassifier(1.0 * RBF(1.0)),
    DecisionTreeClassifier(max_depth=5),
    RandomForestClassifier(max_depth=5, n_estimators=10,
    max_features=1),
    MLPClassifier(alpha=1),
    AdaBoostClassifier(),
    GaussianNB(),
    SVC(kernel = 'linear'),
    SVC(kernel = 'rbf'),
    SVC(kernel = 'sigmoid')
]

models = zip(names, classifiers)

# evaluate each model in turn
results = []
names = []

for name, model in models:
    kfold = model_selection.KFold(n_splits=10, random_state = seed)
    cv_results = model_selection.cross_val_score(model, X_train,
y_train, cv=kfold, scoring=scoring)
    results.append(cv_results)
    names.append(name)
    msg = "%s: %f (%f)" % (name, cv_results.mean(),
cv_results.std())
    print(msg)
```

After running the code, we will get the following output. The `Neural Net` will take a bit longer than the others, as it has the most computational requirements:

```
Nearest Neighbors: 0.823214 (0.113908)
Gaussian Process: 0.873214 (0.056158)
Decision Tree: 0.698214 (0.201628)
Random Forest: 0.607143 (0.162882)

Neural Net: 0.875000 (0.096825)
AdaBoost: 0.925000 (0.114564)
Naive Bayes: 0.837500 (0.137500)
SVM Linear: 0.850000 (0.108972)
SVM RBF: 0.737500 (0.117925)
SVM Sigmoid: 0.569643 (0.159209)
```

Remember that we are running this code on the training data. We don't care about how accurate we can make the data that we're using to fit our algorithm. We care about generalizing to new data, or predicting the results for new instances. This is what makes machine learning algorithms useful.

4. Now, let's test the algorithms on the validation dataset, and print the name, the accuracy score, the classification report for the `y_test` data, and the prediction by running the code snippet:

```
for name, model in models:
    model.fit(X_train, y_train)
    predictions = model.predict(X_test)
    print(name)
    print(accuracy_score(y_test, predictions))
    print(classification_report(y_test, predictions))
```

Upon running this code, we will get meaningful information. Instead of just saying how well our models can fit to the training data, it tells us how well they can actually generalize to new information. We can see that k-nearest neighbors is not actually as effective on the testing data as it is on the training data. The Gaussian Process, though, is doing much better in the 27 cases that we're evaluating on. The `Neural Net` comes in at 92.5%, while the Naive Bayes classifier is at 92%. The support vector machine with a linear kernel, however, actually comes in at 96.296%. Take a look at the following screenshot:

```
Nearest Neighbors                                    AdaBoost
0.7777777777777778                                   0.8518518518518519
              precision    recall  f1-score  support               precision    recall  f1-score  support

          0      1.00       0.65      0.79       17            0      1.00       0.76      0.87       17
          1      0.62       1.00      0.77       10            1      0.71       1.00      0.83       10

avg / total      0.86       0.78      0.78       27   avg / total      0.89       0.85      0.85       27

Gaussian Process                                     Naive Bayes
0.8888888888888888                                   0.9259259259259259
              precision    recall  f1-score  support               precision    recall  f1-score  support

          0      1.00       0.82      0.90       17            0      1.00       0.88      0.94       17
          1      0.77       1.00      0.87       10            1      0.83       1.00      0.91       10

avg / total      0.91       0.89      0.89       27   avg / total      0.94       0.93      0.93       27

Decision Tree                                        SVM Linear
0.7777777777777778                                   0.9629629629629629
              precision    recall  f1-score  support               precision    recall  f1-score  support

          0      1.00       0.65      0.79       17            0      1.00       0.94      0.97       17
          1      0.62       1.00      0.77       10            1      0.91       1.00      0.95       10

avg / total      0.86       0.78      0.78       27   avg / total      0.97       0.96      0.96       27

Random Forest                                        SVM RBF
0.5925925925925926                                   0.7777777777777778
              precision    recall  f1-score  support               precision    recall  f1-score  support

          0      0.88       0.41      0.56       17            0      1.00       0.65      0.79       17
          1      0.47       0.90      0.62       10            1      0.62       1.00      0.77       10

avg / total      0.73       0.59      0.58       27   avg / total      0.86       0.78      0.78       27

Neural Net                                           SVM Sigmoid
0.9259259259259259                                   0.4444444444444444
              precision    recall  f1-score  support               precision    recall  f1-score  support

          0      1.00       0.88      0.94       17            0      1.00       0.12      0.21       17
          1      0.83       1.00      0.91       10            1      0.40       1.00      0.57       10

avg / total      0.94       0.93      0.93       27   avg / total      0.78       0.44      0.34       27
```

While these models did pretty well, it is important to make sure that they can generalize. The AdaBoost classifier actually performed the best, but, once we get down to generalizing to new information, we can see that it is not quite as good. The support vector machine is actually slightly better, in this respect. In the field of bioinformatics, support vector machines are used almost exclusively, so this is, frankly, not that surprising.

Before we wrap this chapter up, let's briefly discuss the output, because this classification report actually gives us a lot of useful information. While we have the avg/total, which is just the ratio of correctly predicted observations to the number of total observations, precision and recall actually give us the most useful information. Precision takes false positives into account; it is actually a ratio of the correctly predicted positive observations against the total predicted positive observations. In the SVM linear kernel, the precision depends on the class. We have 100% precision for the non-promoter class, but the precision is a bit worse for the promoter class.

`recall`, by contrast, takes false negatives into account. It's the ratio of correctly predicted positive observations against all of the observations in the class. The `f1-score` is a weighted average of `precision` and `recall`, so this score takes into account both the false positives and the false negatives. The support, meanwhile, is the number of instances that we had for each. In our case, there are 17 cases that were non-promoters and 10 cases that were promoters. The `f1-score` is probably the best classification metric to use, in this context. We can see that `Neural Net` has the best `f1-score` of any of the classification algorithms that we tried previously. The `Gaussian Process` neural network, and the `Naive Bayes` classifier are also very good.

If you were developing this algorithm for use in a particular application, you'd need to optimize the parameters in the support vector machine with the linear kernel. We could probably improve the results a little bit further by tweaking a few things. A support vector machine doesn't have nearly as many parameters as a neural network, so a neural network would take much longer to optimize. Depending on how much time you have, or how accurate you need your application to be, you can spend time tweaking the different algorithms, to see if you can get better results.

Summary

In this chapter, we were able to predict whether or not a short sequence of E.coli bacteria DNA was a promoter or a non-promoter with 96% accuracy. We looked at how to import data from a repository, and how to convert textual input to numerical data. We then built and trained classification algorithms and compared and contrasted them by using the classification report.

In the next chapter, we will learn about diagnosing coronary artery disease.

Diagnosing Coronary Artery Disease

4

In this chapter, we will be predicting heart disease using neural networks. We will also be looking at a dataset from the UCI repository, which has data on 76 health-related attributes for over 300 patients. We will use this data to predict coronary artery disease. So, if you're looking to get started with machine learning in general—or, more specifically, machine learning applications in the field of healthcare; then this is the project for you.

In this chapter, we will familiarize ourselves with the following topics:

- The dataset
- Fixing missing data
- Splitting the dataset
- Training the neural network
- A comparison of categorical and binary problems

The dataset

To begin with, let's open Command Prompt and execute the following command:

```
cd tutorial
jupyter lab
```

This will take us to the `tutorial` folder. From here, we can open up JupyterLab. This folder is going to be empty right now, but it is where we will be completing this tutorial.

The dataset we're going to use is the heart disease dataset from the UCI repository. You can download this from `archive.ics.uci.edu/ml/machine-learning-databases/heart-disease/`. It has around 303 patients collected from the Cleveland Clinic Foundation. They have also added data from other places as well, but we are only going to look at data from Cleveland for now. If you go over to the `Data` folder, you'll see that we've got lot's of different options:

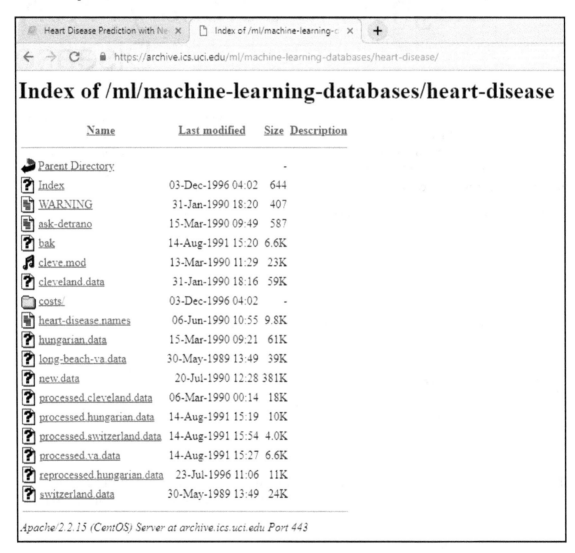

Even if you don't go to the preceding URL, we can directly import all of the files present there directly into our Notebook by downloading them.

The `processed.cleaveland.data` file is the file that we will be using. If we open the `heart-disease.names` file, you'll see more information about the dataset. This information includes the title, source information, past usage, and so on. You will also see different research articles and 14 most commonly used attributes in the research papers that we will be using for this project. So, if you want more information about the dataset, it can be found in the `heart-disease.names` file.

We will now open a default Python Notebook and import all the following libraries, we'll need to work on this project, printing out the versions of each library to make sure we installed the correct ones. To do this, take a look at the following code:

```
import sys
import pandas as pd
import numpy as np
import sklearn
import matplotlib
import keras

print('Python: {}'.format(sys.version))
print('Pandas: {}'.format(pd.__version__))
print('Numpy: {}'.format(np.__version__))
print('Sklearn: {}'.format(sklearn.__version__))
print('Matplotlib: {}'.format(matplotlib.__version__))
print('Keras: {}'.format(keras.__version__))
```

When we run the preceding code snippet, we will get the following output:

```
Python: 2.7.13 |Continuum Analytics, Inc.| (default, May 11 2017, 13:17:26) [MSC v.1500 64 bit (AMD64)]
Pandas: 0.21.0
Numpy: 1.14.3
Sklearn: 0.19.1
Matplotlib: 2.1.0
Keras: 2.1.4
```

Here, you don't need to have exactly the same version numbers, but if you do have different versions installed, then there may be deprecated functions, depending on when you are creating this notebook.

Now we will import some additional packages from the libraries that we need to plot the scatterplot matrix:

```
import matplotlib.pyplot as plt
from pandas.plotting import scatter_matrix
```

Now we will import the dataset and then define the names for each column in our pandas DataFrame. These column names will be the 14 attributes from the `heart-diseases.names` file. We will then read the CSV file from the UCI repository, as follows:

```
# import the heart disease dataset
url =
"http://archive.ics.uci.edu/ml/machine-learning-databases/heart-disease/pro
cessed.cleveland.data"

# the names will be the names of each column in our pandas DataFrame
names = ['age',
 'sex',
 'cp',
 'trestbps',
 'chol',
 'fbs',
 'restecg',
 'thalach',
 'exang',
 'oldpeak',
 'slope',
 'ca',
 'thal',
 'class']

# read the csv
cleveland = pd.read_csv(url, names=names)
```

Now let's print out the shape of the DataFrame, and some additional information with which we can learn more about what we actually just imported and defined:

```
# print the shape of the DataFrame, so we can see how many examples we #
have
print ('Shape of DataFrame: {}'.format(cleveland.shape))
print (cleveland.loc[1])
```

In the following screenshot, we can see that our DataFrame has 303 instances and 14 attributes. We also have an example of a patient with details of the 14 attributes listed:

```
Shape of DataFrame: (303, 14)
age              67
sex               1
cp                4
trestbps        160
chol            286
fbs               0
restecg           2
thalach         108
exang             1
oldpeak         1.5
slope             2
ca              3.0
thal            3.0
class             2
Name: 1, dtype: object
```

The patient in the example is 67 years old, and the sex is 1, which means male (0 is used for female). Furthermore, we can see that he's got some chest pain and suffers from heart disease.

Now, we will print the data for the last 23 patients and examine their details:

```
In [25]:  # print the last twenty or so data points
          cleveland.loc[280:]
```

Out[25]:

	age	sex	cp	trestbps	chol	fbs	restecg	thalach	exang	oldpeak	slope	ca	thal	class
280	57.0	1.0	4.0	110.0	335.0	0.0	0.0	143.0	1.0	3.0	2.0	1.0	7.0	2
281	47.0	1.0	3.0	130.0	253.0	0.0	0.0	179.0	0.0	0.0	1.0	0.0	3.0	0
282	55.0	0.0	4.0	128.0	205.0	0.0	1.0	130.0	1.0	2.0	2.0	1.0	7.0	3
283	35.0	1.0	2.0	122.0	192.0	0.0	0.0	174.0	0.0	0.0	1.0	0.0	3.0	0
284	61.0	1.0	4.0	148.0	203.0	0.0	0.0	161.0	0.0	0.0	1.0	1.0	7.0	2
285	58.0	1.0	4.0	114.0	318.0	0.0	1.0	140.0	0.0	4.4	3.0	3.0	6.0	4
286	58.0	0.0	4.0	170.0	225.0	1.0	2.0	146.0	1.0	2.8	2.0	2.0	6.0	2
287	58.0	1.0	2.0	125.0	220.0	0.0	0.0	144.0	0.0	0.4	2.0	?	7.0	0
288	56.0	1.0	2.0	130.0	221.0	0.0	2.0	163.0	0.0	0.0	1.0	0.0	7.0	0
289	56.0	1.0	2.0	120.0	240.0	0.0	0.0	169.0	0.0	0.0	3.0	0.0	3.0	0
290	67.0	1.0	3.0	152.0	212.0	0.0	2.0	150.0	0.0	0.8	2.0	0.0	7.0	1
291	55.0	0.0	2.0	132.0	342.0	0.0	0.0	166.0	0.0	1.2	1.0	0.0	3.0	0
292	44.0	1.0	4.0	120.0	169.0	0.0	0.0	144.0	1.0	2.8	3.0	0.0	6.0	2
293	63.0	1.0	4.0	140.0	187.0	0.0	2.0	144.0	1.0	4.0	1.0	2.0	7.0	2
294	63.0	0.0	4.0	124.0	197.0	0.0	0.0	136.0	1.0	0.0	2.0	0.0	3.0	1
295	41.0	1.0	2.0	120.0	157.0	0.0	0.0	182.0	0.0	0.0	1.0	0.0	3.0	0
296	59.0	1.0	4.0	164.0	176.0	1.0	2.0	90.0	0.0	1.0	2.0	2.0	6.0	3
297	57.0	0.0	4.0	140.0	241.0	0.0	0.0	123.0	1.0	0.2	2.0	0.0	7.0	1
298	45.0	1.0	1.0	110.0	264.0	0.0	0.0	132.0	0.0	1.2	2.0	0.0	7.0	1
299	68.0	1.0	4.0	144.0	193.0	1.0	0.0	141.0	0.0	3.4	2.0	2.0	7.0	2
300	57.0	1.0	4.0	130.0	131.0	0.0	0.0	115.0	1.0	1.2	2.0	1.0	7.0	3
301	57.0	0.0	2.0	130.0	236.0	0.0	2.0	174.0	0.0	0.0	2.0	1.0	3.0	1
302	38.0	1.0	3.0	138.0	175.0	0.0	0.0	173.0	0.0	0.0	1.0	?	3.0	0

As we can see in the preceding screenshot, we have 14 attributes for each patient, as well as different classifications of heart disease, ranging from 0 to 4. If you actually look at `ca` for patients numbered `287` and `302`, we have question marks here. This means that we have some missing data, which is something we're going to have to handle.

Fixing missing data

Fixing missing data in a dataset is the first important step for a lot of machine learning applications in healthcare, because we're often going to have missing data. There are different ways to handle this, and one of the easiest is to remove those rows entirely. This is especially the case if we're just trying to test a classification algorithm on a neural network, or train one for the first time. This is the route that we are going to take now:

```
In [26]:   # remove missing data (indicated with a "?")
           data = cleveland[~cleveland.isin(['?'])]
           data.loc[280:]
```

Out[26]:

	age	sex	cp	trestbps	chol	fbs	restecg	thalach	exang	oldpeak	slope	ca	thal	class
280	57.0	1.0	4.0	110.0	335.0	0.0	0.0	143.0	1.0	3.0	2.0	1.0	7.0	2
281	47.0	1.0	3.0	130.0	253.0	0.0	0.0	179.0	0.0	0.0	1.0	0.0	3.0	0
282	55.0	0.0	4.0	128.0	205.0	0.0	1.0	130.0	1.0	2.0	2.0	1.0	7.0	3
283	35.0	1.0	2.0	122.0	192.0	0.0	0.0	174.0	0.0	0.0	1.0	0.0	3.0	0
284	61.0	1.0	4.0	148.0	203.0	0.0	0.0	161.0	0.0	0.0	1.0	1.0	7.0	2
285	58.0	1.0	4.0	114.0	318.0	0.0	1.0	140.0	0.0	4.4	3.0	3.0	6.0	4
286	58.0	0.0	4.0	170.0	225.0	1.0	2.0	146.0	1.0	2.8	2.0	2.0	6.0	2
287	58.0	1.0	2.0	125.0	220.0	0.0	0.0	144.0	0.0	0.4	2.0	NaN	7.0	0
288	56.0	1.0	2.0	130.0	221.0	0.0	2.0	163.0	0.0	0.0	1.0	0.0	7.0	0
289	56.0	1.0	2.0	120.0	240.0	0.0	0.0	169.0	0.0	0.0	3.0	0.0	3.0	0
290	67.0	1.0	3.0	152.0	212.0	0.0	2.0	150.0	0.0	0.8	2.0	0.0	7.0	1
291	55.0	0.0	2.0	132.0	342.0	0.0	0.0	166.0	0.0	1.2	1.0	0.0	3.0	0
292	44.0	1.0	4.0	120.0	169.0	0.0	0.0	144.0	1.0	2.8	3.0	0.0	6.0	2
293	63.0	1.0	4.0	140.0	187.0	0.0	2.0	144.0	1.0	4.0	1.0	2.0	7.0	2
294	63.0	0.0	4.0	124.0	197.0	0.0	0.0	136.0	1.0	0.0	2.0	0.0	3.0	1
295	41.0	1.0	2.0	120.0	157.0	0.0	0.0	182.0	0.0	0.0	1.0	0.0	3.0	0
296	59.0	1.0	4.0	164.0	176.0	1.0	2.0	90.0	0.0	1.0	2.0	2.0	6.0	3
297	57.0	0.0	4.0	140.0	241.0	0.0	0.0	123.0	1.0	0.2	2.0	0.0	7.0	1
298	45.0	1.0	1.0	110.0	264.0	0.0	0.0	132.0	0.0	1.2	2.0	0.0	7.0	1
299	68.0	1.0	4.0	144.0	193.0	1.0	0.0	141.0	0.0	3.4	2.0	2.0	7.0	2
300	57.0	1.0	4.0	130.0	131.0	0.0	0.0	115.0	1.0	1.2	2.0	1.0	7.0	3
301	57.0	0.0	2.0	130.0	236.0	0.0	2.0	174.0	0.0	0.0	2.0	1.0	3.0	1
302	38.0	1.0	3.0	138.0	175.0	0.0	0.0	173.0	0.0	0.0	1.0	NaN	3.0	0

We can see, from the data in our new DataFrame, that the question marks have been replaced with NaN. We have nothing in those particular locations. Consequently, we're going to drop the rows with NaN values (or non-number values) from the DataFrame, which is really easy to do with pandas:

```
In [27]:    # drop rows with NaN values from DataFrame
            data = data.dropna(axis=0)
            data.loc[280:]
```

Out[27]:

	age	sex	cp	trestbps	chol	fbs	restecg	thalach	exang	oldpeak	slope	ca	thal	class
280	57.0	1.0	4.0	110.0	335.0	0.0	0.0	143.0	1.0	3.0	2.0	1.0	7.0	2
281	47.0	1.0	3.0	130.0	253.0	0.0	0.0	179.0	0.0	0.0	1.0	0.0	3.0	0
282	55.0	0.0	4.0	128.0	205.0	0.0	1.0	130.0	1.0	2.0	2.0	1.0	7.0	3
283	35.0	1.0	2.0	122.0	192.0	0.0	0.0	174.0	0.0	0.0	1.0	0.0	3.0	0
284	61.0	1.0	4.0	148.0	203.0	0.0	0.0	161.0	0.0	0.0	1.0	1.0	7.0	2
285	58.0	1.0	4.0	114.0	318.0	0.0	1.0	140.0	0.0	4.4	3.0	3.0	6.0	4
286	58.0	0.0	4.0	170.0	225.0	1.0	2.0	146.0	1.0	2.8	2.0	2.0	6.0	2
288	56.0	1.0	2.0	130.0	221.0	0.0	2.0	163.0	0.0	0.0	1.0	0.0	7.0	0
289	56.0	1.0	2.0	120.0	240.0	0.0	0.0	169.0	0.0	0.0	3.0	0.0	3.0	0
290	67.0	1.0	3.0	152.0	212.0	0.0	2.0	150.0	0.0	0.8	2.0	0.0	7.0	1
291	55.0	0.0	2.0	132.0	342.0	0.0	0.0	166.0	0.0	1.2	1.0	0.0	3.0	0
292	44.0	1.0	4.0	120.0	169.0	0.0	0.0	144.0	1.0	2.8	3.0	0.0	6.0	2
293	63.0	1.0	4.0	140.0	187.0	0.0	2.0	144.0	1.0	4.0	1.0	2.0	7.0	2
294	63.0	0.0	4.0	124.0	197.0	0.0	0.0	136.0	1.0	0.0	2.0	0.0	3.0	1
295	41.0	1.0	2.0	120.0	157.0	0.0	0.0	182.0	0.0	0.0	1.0	0.0	3.0	0
296	59.0	1.0	4.0	164.0	176.0	1.0	2.0	90.0	0.0	1.0	2.0	2.0	6.0	3
297	57.0	0.0	4.0	140.0	241.0	0.0	0.0	123.0	1.0	0.2	2.0	0.0	7.0	1
298	45.0	1.0	1.0	110.0	264.0	0.0	0.0	132.0	0.0	1.2	2.0	0.0	7.0	1
299	68.0	1.0	4.0	144.0	193.0	1.0	0.0	141.0	0.0	3.4	2.0	2.0	7.0	2
300	57.0	1.0	4.0	130.0	131.0	0.0	0.0	115.0	1.0	1.2	2.0	1.0	7.0	3
301	57.0	0.0	2.0	130.0	236.0	0.0	2.0	174.0	0.0	0.0	2.0	1.0	3.0	1

In the preceding screenshot, we use the `dropna()` function to drop all the missing data. As we can see, the rows with missing data are gone.

Now let's print the shape again, so that we can see what has happened to our data. How many rows did we lose? We will also print `dtypes` as well, so we know what type of data we have in the dataset:

```
In [28]:  # print the shape and data type of the dataframe
          print data.shape
          print data.dtypes

          (297, 14)
          age           float64
          sex           float64
          cp            float64
          trestbps      float64
          chol          float64
          fbs           float64
          restecg       float64
          thalach       float64
          exang         float64
          oldpeak       float64
          slope         float64
          ca             object
          thal           object
          class          int64
          dtype: object
```

As we can see, we now have 297 instances, so we had 6 patients who didn't have complete data. We still have all 14 of our attributes, and most of them are float values.

We also find that we have some objects. This happens because we had both numerical values and question marks in our last rows, and pandas labeled those as objects. There were both floats and strings included in those. Now we've removed all of the strings, but pandas still has these columns labeled as objects. So what we can do is transform that data back into numerical data. We will tell pandas to treat it all as floats, and then print the datatypes of each column in the dataset:

```
In [29]:  # transform data to numeric to enable further analysis
          data = data.apply(pd.to_numeric)
          data.dtypes

Out[29]:  age        float64
          sex        float64
          cp         float64
          trestbps   float64
          chol       float64
          fbs        float64
          restecg    float64
          thalach    float64
          exang      float64
          oldpeak    float64
          slope      float64
          ca         float64
          thal       float64
          class        int64
          dtype: object
```

So now we can see that we have float values for all columns. Only the class label is going to be an integer.

Now that we have all float values, we can go ahead and print some data characteristics using the built-in describe() function of pandas:

```
In [30]:  # print data characteristics, usings pandas built-in describe() function
          data.describe()
```

Out[30]:	age	sex	cp	trestbps	chol	fbs	restecg	thalach	exang	oldpeak	slope	ca	thal
	297.000000	297.000000	297.000000	297.000000	297.000000	297.000000	297.000000	297.000000	297.000000	297.000000	297.000000	297.000000	297.000000
	54.542088	0.676768	3.158249	131.693603	247.350168	0.144781	0.996633	149.599327	0.326599	1.055556	1.602694	0.676768	4.730640
	9.049736	0.468500	0.964859	17.762806	51.997583	0.352474	0.994914	22.941562	0.469761	1.166123	0.618187	0.938965	1.938629
	29.000000	0.000000	1.000000	94.000000	126.000000	0.000000	0.000000	71.000000	0.000000	0.000000	1.000000	0.000000	3.000000
	48.000000	0.000000	3.000000	120.000000	211.000000	0.000000	0.000000	133.000000	0.000000	0.000000	1.000000	0.000000	3.000000
	56.000000	1.000000	3.000000	130.000000	243.000000	0.000000	1.000000	153.000000	0.000000	0.800000	2.000000	0.000000	3.000000
	61.000000	1.000000	4.000000	140.000000	276.000000	0.000000	2.000000	166.000000	1.000000	1.600000	2.000000	1.000000	7.000000
	77.000000	1.000000	4.000000	200.000000	564.000000	1.000000	2.000000	202.000000	1.000000	6.200000	3.000000	3.000000	7.000000

As we can see, we have all sorts of information about each attribute—297 instances for each of them. This includes mean, std, min, the Q1, Q2, and Q3 quartiles, and max, for all of the different attributes in our dataset. Again, remember that it's really important to explore your data before trying to apply machine learning algorithms. This is because, depending on your data, you're going to lean towards or away from different techniques. So, if all of your data is numerical, then that will be best for a regression problem. If you have categorical data, classification is a better option than regression. In our case, we can use all of these for a classification problem with our neural network. In some situations, you might have to normalize the data, but this won't always be necessary.

One more convenient thing we can do is plot histograms for each variable. We will plot histograms using the `data.hist()` function, and then run `plt.show()`, which will print the histograms, as seen in the following screenshot:

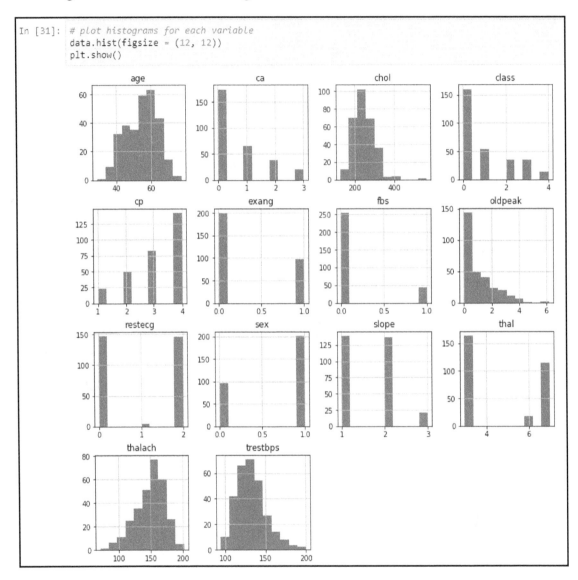

As we can see, some of the histograms have continuous numerical bars, whereas others have more categorical labels. Also, we have `class` up in the upper right-hand corner. It looks like they're just organized alphabetically, and that is just fine. One thing to note here is that we have just over 150 patients that didn't have heart disease. They had a label of 0 for the `class` label. We also had a decreasing number of patients with more severe levels of heart disease, where number 4 represents the most severe form of heart disease—we have the fewest patients for this. As we know that we have around 300 patients in our dataset, we can say that we have a pretty even split between patients without heart disease and patients with heart disease, which is actually good for our particular application.

Splitting the dataset

Now we will split our dataset into training and testing datasets. We're going to use sklearn's `train_test_split` function to generate a training dataset, which will be about 80% of the total data, and then a testing dataset, which will be 20% of the total data. The class values in this dataset contain multiple types of heart disease, with values ranging from 0 (healthy) to 4 (severe heart disease). Consequently, we will convert our class data into categorical labels.

Let's create X and y datasets for training. So, first, we want to split our class label into its own y value. We will import the `model_selection` package from sklearn and convert the X DataFrame to a NumPy array, taking everything but the `class` attribute. Likewise, for the y DataFrame, we will convert this into a NumPy array, but here we will only take the `class` attribute. Then, we will randomly split the DataFrames into training and testing datasets, using the `train_test_split()` function:

```
# create X and Y datasets for training
from sklearn import model_selection

X = np.array(data.drop(['class'], 1))
y = np.array(data['class'])

X_train, X_test, y_train, y_test = model_selection.train_test_split(X, y,
test_size = 0.2)
```

Now we will convert the data into categorical labels. To do so, we will import `to_categorical` from `keras.utils.np_utils` and convert `y_train` to `Y_train` and `y_test` to `Y_test`, printing the shape and the first 10 instances:

```
In [33]:   # convert the data to categorical labels
           from keras.utils.np_utils import to_categorical

           Y_train = to_categorical(y_train, num_classes=None)
           Y_test = to_categorical(y_test, num_classes=None)
           print Y_train.shape
           print Y_train[:10]

           (237L, 5L)
           [[0. 0. 0. 0. 1.]
            [0. 0. 0. 0. 1.]
            [1. 0. 0. 0. 0.]
            [0. 0. 1. 0. 0.]
            [1. 0. 0. 0. 0.]
            [0. 0. 1. 0. 0.]
            [0. 1. 0. 0. 0.]
            [1. 0. 0. 0. 0.]
            [0. 1. 0. 0. 0.]
            [1. 0. 0. 0. 0.]]
```

As we can see in the preceding image, we have `(237L, 5L)` as the shape of our data. This is the number of patients in our training dataset, and we now have categorical labels. These are one-hot encoded vectors. So, instead of a 0 in the first row, the index 0 in this short vector has a 1; everything else is a 0. The second row is going to be a 2, as it has a 1 in the third location. Those are our categorical labels, which are also, importantly, the type of label that Keras is going to need for our neural network.

Training the neural network

Now, we will move on to building and training the neural network. To do so, let's import some specific layers from Keras. Then, we will define a `create_model()` function to build the Keras model, and define the model type as `Sequential`. After this, we will define an input layer, a hidden layer and an output layer, compile the model, and finally print the model:

```
In [34]: from keras.models import Sequential
         from keras.layers import Dense
         from keras.optimizers import Adam

         # define a function to build the keras model
         def create_model():
             # create model
             model = Sequential()
             model.add(Dense(8, input_dim=13, kernel_initializer='normal', activation='relu'))
             model.add(Dense(4, kernel_initializer='normal', activation='relu'))
             model.add(Dense(5, activation='softmax'))

             # compile model
             adam = Adam(lr=0.001)
             model.compile(loss='categorical_crossentropy', optimizer=adam, metrics=['accuracy'])
             return model

         model = create_model()

         print(model.summary())

         _____
         Layer (type)                 Output Shape              Param #
         =================================================================
         dense_7 (Dense)              (None, 8)                 112
         _____
         dense_8 (Dense)              (None, 4)                 36
         _____
         dense_9 (Dense)              (None, 5)                 25
         =================================================================
         Total params: 173
         Trainable params: 173
         Non-trainable params: 0
         _____
         None
```

As we see in the preceding screenshot, we have our model summary. We have 112 parameters for the first layer, 36 for the second, and 25 for the third layer. We have a total of 173 parameters. These are all trainable data for our neural network, which is what we will be using to classify the patients as either having coronary artery disease or not having coronary artery disease.

We will now fit the model to the training data using the `model.fit()` function:

```
In [38]: # fit the model to the training data
         model.fit(X_train, Y_train, epochs=100, batch_size=10, verbose = 1)

Epoch 1/100
237/237 [==============================] - 0s 207us/step - loss: 1.6193 - acc: 0.2911
Epoch 2/100
237/237 [==============================] - 0s 194us/step - loss: 1.5907 - acc: 0.5190
Epoch 3/100
237/237 [==============================] - 0s 287us/step - loss: 1.5769 - acc: 0.5190
Epoch 4/100
237/237 [==============================] - 0s 148us/step - loss: 1.5636 - acc: 0.5232
Epoch 5/100
237/237 [==============================] - 0s 152us/step - loss: 1.5498 - acc: 0.5232
Epoch 6/100
237/237 [==============================] - 0s 148us/step - loss: 1.5360 - acc: 0.5232
Epoch 7/100
237/237 [==============================] - 0s 122us/step - loss: 1.5216 - acc: 0.5232
Epoch 8/100
237/237 [==============================] - 0s 169us/step - loss: 1.5075 - acc: 0.5232
Epoch 9/100
237/237 [==============================] - 0s 135us/step - loss: 1.4930 - acc: 0.5232
Epoch 10/100
237/237 [==============================] - 0s 122us/step - loss: 1.4795 - acc: 0.5232
Epoch 11/100
237/237 [==============================] - 0s 143us/step - loss: 1.4659 - acc: 0.5232
Epoch 12/100
237/237 [==============================] - 0s 143us/step - loss: 1.4525 - acc: 0.5232
Epoch 13/100
237/237 [==============================] - 0s 169us/step - loss: 1.4401 - acc: 0.5232
Epoch 14/100
237/237 [==============================] - 0s 127us/step - loss: 1.4273 - acc: 0.5232
Epoch 15/100
237/237 [==============================] - 0s 135us/step - loss: 1.4158 - acc: 0.5232
Epoch 16/100
237/237 [==============================] - 0s 131us/step - loss: 1.4042 - acc: 0.5232
Epoch 17/100
237/237 [==============================] - 0s 131us/step - loss: 1.3744 - acc: 0.5232
Epoch 18/100
237/237 [==============================] - 0s 131us/step - loss: 1.3500 - acc: 0.5232
Epoch 19/100
237/237 [==============================] - 0s 131us/step - loss: 1.3297 - acc: 0.5232
Epoch 20/100
237/237 [==============================] - 0s 118us/step - loss: 1.3110 - acc: 0.5232
Epoch 21/100
237/237 [==============================] - 0s 127us/step - loss: 1.2928 - acc: 0.5232
Epoch 22/100
237/237 [==============================] - 0s 139us/step - loss: 1.2766 - acc: 0.5232
Epoch 23/100
237/237 [==============================] - 0s 143us/step - loss: 1.2575 - acc: 0.5232
Epoch 24/100
237/237 [==============================] - 0s 127us/step - loss: 1.2670 - acc: 0.5232
Epoch 25/100
237/237 [==============================] - 0s 122us/step - loss: 1.2401 - acc: 0.5232
Epoch 26/100
237/237 [==============================] - 0s 127us/step - loss: 1.2307 - acc: 0.5232
Epoch 27/100
237/237 [==============================] - 0s 152us/step - loss: 1.2155 - acc: 0.5232
Epoch 28/100
237/237 [==============================] - 0s 177us/step - loss: 1.2265 - acc: 0.5232
Epoch 29/100
237/237 [==============================] - 0s 148us/step - loss: 1.2047 - acc: 0.5232
Epoch 30/100
237/237 [==============================] - 0s 148us/step - loss: 1.1927 - acc: 0.5232
Epoch 31/100
237/237 [==============================] - 0s 156us/step - loss: 1.1792 - acc: 0.5232
Epoch 32/100
237/237 [==============================] - 0s 156us/step - loss: 1.1733 - acc: 0.5232
Epoch 33/100
237/237 [==============================] - 0s 139us/step - loss: 1.1600 - acc: 0.5232
Epoch 34/100
237/237 [==============================] - 0s 143us/step - loss: 1.1714 - acc: 0.5232
Epoch 35/100
237/237 [==============================] - 0s 127us/step - loss: 1.1578 - acc: 0.5232
Epoch 36/100
237/237 [==============================] - 0s 135us/step - loss: 1.1525 - acc: 0.5232
Epoch 37/100
237/237 [==============================] - 0s 131us/step - loss: 1.1510 - acc: 0.5232
Epoch 38/100
237/237 [==============================] - 0s 148us/step - loss: 1.1371 - acc: 0.5232
Epoch 39/100
237/237 [==============================] - 0s 143us/step - loss: 1.1405 - acc: 0.5232
Epoch 40/100
237/237 [==============================] - 0s 135us/step - loss: 1.1256 - acc: 0.5232
Epoch 41/100
237/237 [==============================] - 0s 148us/step - loss: 1.1302 - acc: 0.5232
Epoch 42/100
237/237 [==============================] - 0s 135us/step - loss: 1.1241 - acc: 0.5232
Epoch 43/100
237/237 [==============================] - 0s 127us/step - loss: 1.1065 - acc: 0.5232
Epoch 44/100
237/237 [==============================] - 0s 148us/step - loss: 1.1146 - acc: 0.5232
Epoch 45/100
237/237 [==============================] - 0s 143us/step - loss: 1.1051 - acc: 0.5232
Epoch 46/100
237/237 [==============================] - 0s 135us/step - loss: 1.0943 - acc: 0.5232
Epoch 47/100
237/237 [==============================] - 0s 118us/step - loss: 1.1030 - acc: 0.5232
Epoch 48/100
237/237 [==============================] - 0s 127us/step - loss: 1.0912 - acc: 0.5232
Epoch 49/100
237/237 [==============================] - 0s 131us/step - loss: 1.0771 - acc: 0.5232
Epoch 50/100
237/237 [==============================] - 0s 127us/step - loss: 1.0775 - acc: 0.5232
Epoch 51/100
237/237 [==============================] - 0s 110us/step - loss: 1.0839 - acc: 0.5232
Epoch 52/100
237/237 [==============================] - 0s 135us/step - loss: 1.0798 - acc: 0.5232
Epoch 53/100
237/237 [==============================] - 0s 127us/step - loss: 1.0951 - acc: 0.5232
Epoch 54/100
237/237 [==============================] - 0s 139us/step - loss: 1.0738 - acc: 0.5443
Epoch 55/100
237/237 [==============================] - 0s 118us/step - loss: 1.0589 - acc: 0.5612
Epoch 56/100
237/237 [==============================] - 0s 131us/step - loss: 1.0499 - acc: 0.5443
Epoch 57/100
237/237 [==============================] - 0s 127us/step - loss: 1.0418 - acc: 0.5485
Epoch 58/100
237/237 [==============================] - 0s 131us/step - loss: 1.0461 - acc: 0.5485
Epoch 59/100
237/237 [==============================] - 0s 122us/step - loss: 1.0387 - acc: 0.5654
Epoch 60/100
237/237 [==============================] - 0s 148us/step - loss: 1.0329 - acc: 0.5654
Epoch 61/100
237/237 [==============================] - 0s 131us/step - loss: 1.0409 - acc: 0.5570
Epoch 62/100
237/237 [==============================] - 0s 131us/step - loss: 1.0312 - acc: 0.5654
Epoch 63/100
237/237 [==============================] - 0s 131us/step - loss: 1.0231 - acc: 0.5654
Epoch 64/100
237/237 [==============================] - 0s 143us/step - loss: 1.0203 - acc: 0.5612
Epoch 65/100
237/237 [==============================] - 0s 122us/step - loss: 1.0137 - acc: 0.5612
Epoch 66/100
237/237 [==============================] - 0s 118us/step - loss: 1.0165 - acc: 0.5527
Epoch 67/100
237/237 [==============================] - 0s 131us/step - loss: 1.0076 - acc: 0.5612
Epoch 68/100
237/237 [==============================] - 0s 114us/step - loss: 1.0124 - acc: 0.5612
Epoch 69/100
237/237 [==============================] - 0s 127us/step - loss: 1.0116 - acc: 0.5696
Epoch 70/100
237/237 [==============================] - 0s 122us/step - loss: 1.0068 - acc: 0.5570
Epoch 71/100
237/237 [==============================] - 0s 143us/step - loss: 1.0017 - acc: 0.5696
Epoch 72/100
237/237 [==============================] - 0s 127us/step - loss: 0.9954 - acc: 0.5696
Epoch 73/100
237/237 [==============================] - 0s 110us/step - loss: 1.0066 - acc: 0.5612
Epoch 74/100
237/237 [==============================] - 0s 122us/step - loss: 0.9907 - acc: 0.5654
Epoch 75/100
237/237 [==============================] - 0s 122us/step - loss: 0.9897 - acc: 0.5612
Epoch 76/100
237/237 [==============================] - 0s 118us/step - loss: 0.9926 - acc: 0.5612
Epoch 77/100
237/237 [==============================] - 0s 118us/step - loss: 0.9854 - acc: 0.5654
Epoch 78/100
237/237 [==============================] - 0s 131us/step - loss: 0.9770 - acc: 0.5738
Epoch 79/100
237/237 [==============================] - 0s 127us/step - loss: 0.9727 - acc: 0.5696
Epoch 80/100
237/237 [==============================] - 0s 135us/step - loss: 0.9837 - acc: 0.5781
Epoch 81/100
237/237 [==============================] - 0s 122us/step - loss: 0.9702 - acc: 0.5696
Epoch 82/100
237/237 [==============================] - 0s 135us/step - loss: 0.9671 - acc: 0.5654
Epoch 83/100
237/237 [==============================] - 0s 118us/step - loss: 0.9734 - acc: 0.5612
Epoch 84/100
237/237 [==============================] - 0s 122us/step - loss: 0.9641 - acc: 0.5696
Epoch 85/100
237/237 [==============================] - 0s 105us/step - loss: 0.9616 - acc: 0.5612
Epoch 86/100
237/237 [==============================] - 0s 122us/step - loss: 0.9616 - acc: 0.5781
Epoch 87/100
237/237 [==============================] - 0s 135us/step - loss: 0.9582 - acc: 0.5696
Epoch 88/100
237/237 [==============================] - 0s 122us/step - loss: 0.9552 - acc: 0.5696
Epoch 89/100
237/237 [==============================] - 0s 118us/step - loss: 0.9630 - acc: 0.5907
Epoch 90/100
237/237 [==============================] - 0s 122us/step - loss: 0.9506 - acc: 0.6076
Epoch 91/100
237/237 [==============================] - 0s 118us/step - loss: 0.9559 - acc: 0.6287
Epoch 92/100
237/237 [==============================] - 0s 127us/step - loss: 0.9597 - acc: 0.6203
Epoch 93/100
237/237 [==============================] - 0s 127us/step - loss: 0.9535 - acc: 0.6245
Epoch 94/100
237/237 [==============================] - 0s 135us/step - loss: 0.9604 - acc: 0.5992
Epoch 95/100
237/237 [==============================] - 0s 139us/step - loss: 0.9460 - acc: 0.6076
Epoch 96/100
237/237 [==============================] - 0s 148us/step - loss: 0.9559 - acc: 0.6287
Epoch 97/100
237/237 [==============================] - 0s 135us/step - loss: 0.9387 - acc: 0.6160
Epoch 98/100
237/237 [==============================] - 0s 114us/step - loss: 0.9416 - acc: 0.6245
Epoch 99/100
237/237 [==============================] - 0s 135us/step - loss: 0.9375 - acc: 0.6160
Epoch 100/100
237/237 [==============================] - 0s 122us/step - loss: 0.9383 - acc: 0.6160

<keras.callbacks.History at 0x17ac65c0>
```

From the preceding screenshot, we see that the model prints out a loss value for each epoch. We can also see that we're at between 59% accuracy and 61% accuracy for the later epochs. This is our categorical result, but what we're actually looking for is how we can improve these results using a simple binary classification problem. We had 5 classes: 0 (healthy); and then 1 through 4 for different levels of heart disease. What if we just say whether or not the patient is healthy or at risk of heart disease? We will convert the data to two classes: 0 and 1, and we'll see how much that actually improves our results. Then we will compare and contrast our categorical results and our binary results at the end.

To convert this into a binary classification problem to identify the presence of any degree of heart disease or not, we will copy the Y_train and the Y_test and set to it to Y_train_binary and Y_test_binary respectively; then, any data whose value is greater than 0 will be converted to 1, while all the zeros will stay as 0. We will then print the first 20 patients' data:

```
In [36]:  # convert into binary classification problem - heart disease or no heart disease
          Y_train_binary = y_train.copy()
          Y_test_binary = y_test.copy()

          Y_train_binary[Y_train_binary > 0] = 1
          Y_test_binary[Y_test_binary > 0] = 1

          print Y_train_binary[:20]

          [1 1 0 1 0 1 1 0 1 0 0 1 0 1 0 0 0 0 0 1]
```

So now, we have our values reading 0 and 1, but no longer have different levels of heart disease. Now all we have is *healthy*, represented by 0; or *at risk of heart disease*, represented by 1. This is a binary classification problem.

A comparison of categorical and binary problems

We will compare and contrast our categorical classification problem and the binary classification problem just covered. To do this, first we have to create a new model, since we've changed our data. We will define a binary model, then we will define an input layer, a hidden layer and an output layer, compile the model, and finally print the model:

```
In [37]:  # define a new keras model for binary classification
          def create_binary_model():
              # create model
              model = Sequential()
              model.add(Dense(8, input_dim=13, kernel_initializer='normal', activation='relu'))
              model.add(Dense(4, kernel_initializer='normal', activation='relu'))
              model.add(Dense(1, activation='sigmoid'))

              # Compile model
              adam = Adam(lr=0.001)
              model.compile(loss='binary_crossentropy', optimizer=adam, metrics=['accuracy'])
              return model

          binary_model = create_binary_model()

          print(binary_model.summary())
```

Layer (type)	Output Shape	Param #
dense_10 (Dense)	(None, 8)	112
dense_11 (Dense)	(None, 4)	36
dense_12 (Dense)	(None, 1)	5

```
Total params: 153
Trainable params: 153
Non-trainable params: 0
```

```
None
```

As we see in the screenshot, our third layer has only one output value, so it's going to be 0 and 1, instead of a one-hot encoded vector for a categorical classification. So, our binary model is ready, and now we're in the training phase—let's fit the binary model to our binary data that we curated:

```
In [38]: # fit the binary model on the training data
         binary_model.fit(X_train, Y_train_binary, epochs=100, batch_size=10, verbose = 1)
```

```
Epoch 1/100
237/237 [==============================] - 0s 460us/step - loss: 0.7973 - acc: 0.4979
Epoch 2/100
237/237 [==============================] - 0s 557us/step - loss: 0.6848 - acc: 0.6203
Epoch 3/100
237/237 [==============================] - 0s 549us/step - loss: 0.6543 - acc: 0.6118
Epoch 4/100
237/237 [==============================] - 0s 599us/step - loss: 0.6367 - acc: 0.6879
Epoch 5/100
237/237 [==============================] - 0s 675us/step - loss: 0.6313 - acc: 0.6624
Epoch 6/100
237/237 [==============================] - 0s 633us/step - loss: 0.6231 - acc: 0.6835
Epoch 7/100
237/237 [==============================] - 0s 443us/step - loss: 0.6170 - acc: 0.6540
Epoch 8/100
237/237 [==============================] - 0s 549us/step - loss: 0.6207 - acc: 0.6667
Epoch 9/100
237/237 [==============================] - 0s 684us/step - loss: 0.5848 - acc: 0.7257
Epoch 10/100
237/237 [==============================] - 0s 612us/step - loss: 0.5958 - acc: 0.6835
Epoch 11/100
237/237 [==============================] - 0s 700us/step - loss: 0.5761 - acc: 0.7089
Epoch 12/100
237/237 [==============================] - 0s 570us/step - loss: 0.5664 - acc: 0.7215
Epoch 13/100
237/237 [==============================] - 0s 616us/step - loss: 0.5537 - acc: 0.7426
Epoch 14/100
237/237 [==============================] - 0s 654us/step - loss: 0.5439 - acc: 0.7342
Epoch 15/100
237/237 [==============================] - 0s 553us/step - loss: 0.5492 - acc: 0.7426
Epoch 16/100
237/237 [==============================] - 0s 540us/step - loss: 0.5340 - acc: 0.7553
Epoch 17/100
237/237 [==============================] - 0s 456us/step - loss: 0.5244 - acc: 0.7426
Epoch 18/100
237/237 [==============================] - 0s 586us/step - loss: 0.5155 - acc: 0.7468
Epoch 19/100
237/237 [==============================] - 0s 578us/step - loss: 0.5069 - acc: 0.7764
Epoch 20/100
237/237 [==============================] - 0s 574us/step - loss: 0.5043 - acc: 0.7384
Epoch 21/100
237/237 [==============================] - 0s 574us/step - loss: 0.4952 - acc: 0.7848
Epoch 22/100
237/237 [==============================] - 0s 582us/step - loss: 0.4962 - acc: 0.7511
Epoch 23/100
237/237 [==============================] - 0s 540us/step - loss: 0.4840 - acc: 0.7595
Epoch 24/100
237/237 [==============================] - 0s 679us/step - loss: 0.5205 - acc: 0.7300
Epoch 25/100
237/237 [==============================] - 0s 418us/step - loss: 0.4855 - acc: 0.7722

Epoch 51/100
237/237 [==============================] - 0s 228us/step - loss: 0.3812 - acc: 0.8439
Epoch 52/100
237/237 [==============================] - 0s 228us/step - loss: 0.3880 - acc: 0.8312
Epoch 53/100
237/237 [==============================] - 0s 232us/step - loss: 0.3676 - acc: 0.8692
Epoch 54/100
237/237 [==============================] - 0s 207us/step - loss: 0.3716 - acc: 0.8565
Epoch 55/100
237/237 [==============================] - 0s 232us/step - loss: 0.3591 - acc: 0.8734
Epoch 56/100
237/237 [==============================] - 0s 215us/step - loss: 0.3625 - acc: 0.8565
Epoch 57/100
237/237 [==============================] - 0s 232us/step - loss: 0.3587 - acc: 0.8692
Epoch 58/100
237/237 [==============================] - 0s 236us/step - loss: 0.3604 - acc: 0.8861
Epoch 59/100
237/237 [==============================] - 0s 236us/step - loss: 0.3599 - acc: 0.8692
Epoch 60/100
237/237 [==============================] - 0s 207us/step - loss: 0.3513 - acc: 0.8776
Epoch 61/100
237/237 [==============================] - 0s 367us/step - loss: 0.3853 - acc: 0.8650
Epoch 62/100
237/237 [==============================] - 0s 283us/step - loss: 0.3820 - acc: 0.8439
Epoch 63/100
237/237 [==============================] - 0s 215us/step - loss: 0.4204 - acc: 0.8397
Epoch 64/100
237/237 [==============================] - 0s 312us/step - loss: 0.3694 - acc: 0.8523
Epoch 65/100
237/237 [==============================] - 0s 236us/step - loss: 0.3592 - acc: 0.8692
Epoch 66/100
237/237 [==============================] - 0s 219us/step - loss: 0.3523 - acc: 0.8692
Epoch 67/100
237/237 [==============================] - 0s 291us/step - loss: 0.3566 - acc: 0.8692
Epoch 68/100
237/237 [==============================] - 0s 211us/step - loss: 0.3705 - acc: 0.8270
Epoch 69/100
237/237 [==============================] - 0s 241us/step - loss: 0.3562 - acc: 0.8608
Epoch 70/100
237/237 [==============================] - 0s 203us/step - loss: 0.3765 - acc: 0.8692
Epoch 71/100
237/237 [==============================] - 0s 219us/step - loss: 0.3564 - acc: 0.8650
Epoch 72/100
237/237 [==============================] - 0s 215us/step - loss: 0.3719 - acc: 0.8650
Epoch 73/100
237/237 [==============================] - 0s 198us/step - loss: 0.3559 - acc: 0.8565
Epoch 74/100
237/237 [==============================] - 0s 224us/step - loss: 0.3601 - acc: 0.8523
Epoch 75/100
237/237 [==============================] - 0s 190us/step - loss: 0.3533 - acc: 0.8608
```

```
Epoch 26/100
237/237 [==============================] - 0s 384us/step - loss: 0.4735 - acc: 0.7764
Epoch 27/100
237/237 [==============================] - 0s 494us/step - loss: 0.4619 - acc: 0.7975
Epoch 28/100
237/237 [==============================] - 0s 367us/step - loss: 0.4504 - acc: 0.8017
Epoch 29/100
237/237 [==============================] - 0s 316us/step - loss: 0.4520 - acc: 0.7975
Epoch 30/100
237/237 [==============================] - 0s 338us/step - loss: 0.4446 - acc: 0.8228
Epoch 31/100
237/237 [==============================] - 0s 312us/step - loss: 0.4422 - acc: 0.8059
Epoch 32/100
237/237 [==============================] - 0s 333us/step - loss: 0.4353 - acc: 0.8101
Epoch 33/100
237/237 [==============================] - 0s 354us/step - loss: 0.4240 - acc: 0.8059
Epoch 34/100
237/237 [==============================] - 0s 338us/step - loss: 0.4628 - acc: 0.7806
Epoch 35/100
237/237 [==============================] - 0s 376us/step - loss: 0.4130 - acc: 0.8143
Epoch 36/100
237/237 [==============================] - 0s 312us/step - loss: 0.4077 - acc: 0.8186
Epoch 37/100
237/237 [==============================] - 0s 304us/step - loss: 0.4256 - acc: 0.8101
Epoch 38/100
237/237 [==============================] - 0s 333us/step - loss: 0.4041 - acc: 0.8270
Epoch 39/100
237/237 [==============================] - 0s 312us/step - loss: 0.4030 - acc: 0.8439
Epoch 40/100
237/237 [==============================] - 0s 295us/step - loss: 0.3976 - acc: 0.8397
Epoch 41/100
237/237 [==============================] - 0s 304us/step - loss: 0.3996 - acc: 0.8270
Epoch 42/100
237/237 [==============================] - 0s 300us/step - loss: 0.4314 - acc: 0.7932
Epoch 43/100
237/237 [==============================] - 0s 291us/step - loss: 0.3902 - acc: 0.8439
Epoch 44/100
237/237 [==============================] - 0s 287us/step - loss: 0.3980 - acc: 0.8481
Epoch 45/100
237/237 [==============================] - 0s 346us/step - loss: 0.3850 - acc: 0.8312
Epoch 46/100
237/237 [==============================] - 0s 291us/step - loss: 0.3873 - acc: 0.8565
Epoch 47/100
237/237 [==============================] - 0s 228us/step - loss: 0.3728 - acc: 0.8565
Epoch 48/100
237/237 [==============================] - 0s 232us/step - loss: 0.4108 - acc: 0.8312
Epoch 49/100
237/237 [==============================] - 0s 295us/step - loss: 0.3728 - acc: 0.8650
Epoch 50/100
237/237 [==============================] - 0s 232us/step - loss: 0.3721 - acc: 0.8565

Epoch 76/100
237/237 [==============================] - 0s 207us/step - loss: 0.3598 - acc: 0.8734
Epoch 77/100
237/237 [==============================] - 0s 194us/step - loss: 0.3506 - acc: 0.8650
Epoch 78/100
237/237 [==============================] - 0s 186us/step - loss: 0.4006 - acc: 0.8734
Epoch 79/100
237/237 [==============================] - 0s 203us/step - loss: 0.3521 - acc: 0.8565
Epoch 80/100
237/237 [==============================] - 0s 215us/step - loss: 0.3677 - acc: 0.8734
Epoch 81/100
237/237 [==============================] - 0s 274us/step - loss: 0.3466 - acc: 0.8565
Epoch 82/100
237/237 [==============================] - 0s 203us/step - loss: 0.4005 - acc: 0.8228
Epoch 83/100
237/237 [==============================] - 0s 219us/step - loss: 0.3642 - acc: 0.8592
Epoch 84/100
237/237 [==============================] - 0s 215us/step - loss: 0.3394 - acc: 0.8692
Epoch 85/100
237/237 [==============================] - 0s 203us/step - loss: 0.3484 - acc: 0.8734
Epoch 86/100
237/237 [==============================] - 0s 224us/step - loss: 0.3529 - acc: 0.8650
Epoch 87/100
237/237 [==============================] - 0s 207us/step - loss: 0.3528 - acc: 0.8650
Epoch 88/100
237/237 [==============================] - 0s 203us/step - loss: 0.3473 - acc: 0.8734
Epoch 89/100
237/237 [==============================] - 0s 198us/step - loss: 0.3509 - acc: 0.8565
Epoch 90/100
237/237 [==============================] - 0s 194us/step - loss: 0.3390 - acc: 0.8734
Epoch 91/100
237/237 [==============================] - 0s 207us/step - loss: 0.3598 - acc: 0.8481
Epoch 92/100
237/237 [==============================] - 0s 219us/step - loss: 0.3503 - acc: 0.8608
Epoch 93/100
237/237 [==============================] - 0s 190us/step - loss: 0.3492 - acc: 0.8608
Epoch 94/100
237/237 [==============================] - 0s 211us/step - loss: 0.3719 - acc: 0.8565
Epoch 95/100
237/237 [==============================] - 0s 207us/step - loss: 0.3495 - acc: 0.8650
Epoch 96/100
237/237 [==============================] - 0s 181us/step - loss: 0.3465 - acc: 0.8734
Epoch 97/100
237/237 [==============================] - 0s 203us/step - loss: 0.3582 - acc: 0.8608
Epoch 98/100
237/237 [==============================] - 0s 198us/step - loss: 0.3476 - acc: 0.8734
Epoch 99/100
237/237 [==============================] - 0s 295us/step - loss: 0.3432 - acc: 0.8523
Epoch 100/100
237/237 [==============================] - 0s 215us/step - loss: 0.3385 - acc: 0.8776

<keras.callbacks.History at 0x17200e48>
```

As we can see in the preceding screenshot, we're getting better accuracy than we were on our categorical classification problem. Binary classification is like a multiple-choice question with A or B as choices, and our categorical problem is a multiple-choice question with A, B, C, D, E, and F as the choices.

Now, we will do some actual performance metrics on our testing dataset, so that we can see what our results actually mean and what we're actually predicting in each of these cases. We will generate a classification report using predictions for the categorical model, and then we'll do the same for the binary model as well. To do this, we will need the `sklearn.metrics` function. We will import the `classification_report` function and the `accuracy_score` function. To make predictions with the Keras model in categorical prediction, we will call `categorical_pred` and print the result:

```
In [26]:  # generate classification report using predictions for categorical model
          from sklearn.metrics import classification_report, accuracy_score

          categorical_pred = model.predict(X_test)

In [27]:  categorical_pred

Out[27]:  array([[1.01122111e-01, 2.55058527e-01, 2.35597149e-01, 3.12478006e-01,
          9.57441553e-02],
          [5.33457756e-01, 2.98719645e-01, 9.35494676e-02, 5.82468845e-02,
          1.60261374e-02],
          [5.80684125e-01, 2.97834665e-01, 7.01721087e-02, 4.20845188e-02,
          9.22461320e-03],
          [1.16159856e-01, 2.39220947e-01, 2.43541703e-01, 2.89612323e-01,
          1.11465104e-01],
          [1.20953463e-01, 2.34275043e-01, 2.45628655e-01, 2.82606691e-01,
          1.16536178e-01],
          [1.21686250e-01, 2.33523130e-01, 2.45929852e-01, 2.81546861e-01,
          1.17313892e-01],
          [6.76299691e-01, 2.52068818e-01, 4.43583280e-02, 2.27026902e-02,
          4.57041990e-03],
          [1.95704728e-01, 3.10539395e-01, 2.08661154e-01, 2.19161719e-01,
          6.59330785e-02],
          [3.60710382e-01, 3.46726894e-01, 1.44093186e-01, 1.18074283e-01,
          3.03952657e-02],
          [1.15559876e-01, 2.39843398e-01, 2.43266031e-01, 2.90498316e-01,
          1.10832416e-01],
          [8.28893661e-01, 1.49000451e-01, 1.55386953e-02, 5.51294256e-03,
          1.05435983e-03],
          [1.06301658e-01, 2.49546438e-01, 2.38584325e-01, 3.04440856e-01,
          1.01126775e-01],
          [4.37164307e-01, 3.19904685e-01, 1.26573503e-01, 9.00377557e-02,
          2.63197385e-02],
          [6.83460057e-01, 2.45263875e-01, 4.43375707e-02, 2.22279448e-02,
          4.71051177e-03],
          [6.97706223e-01, 2.37085029e-01, 4.10035960e-02, 2.00037956e-02,
          4.20142151e-03],
          [6.39340281e-01, 2.71579951e-01, 5.36735281e-02, 2.93161590e-02,
          6.09008828e-03],
          [3.31699371e-01, 3.50276917e-01, 1.53014556e-01, 1.31520733e-01,
          3.34884711e-02],
          [1.06818460e-01, 2.48999819e-01, 2.38867462e-01, 3.03648621e-01,
          1.01665713e-01],
          [6.94831192e-01, 2.40902245e-01, 4.03533690e-02, 1.99141204e-02,
          3.99902463e-03],
          [8.40716958e-01, 1.41284823e-01, 1.28218718e-02, 4.40968201e-03,
          7.66728190e-04],
          [9.30293977e-01, 6.61148280e-02, 2.85831373e-03, 6.40276470e-04,
          9.25873755e-05],
          [8.31946492e-01, 1.46950290e-01, 1.48829427e-02, 5.23659727e-03,
          9.83754406e-04],
          [1.70788392e-01, 3.06327462e-01, 2.14115247e-01, 2.39519149e-01,
          6.92496821e-02],
          [9.06477571e-01, 8.70160535e-02, 5.00054751e-03, 1.30012271e-03,
          2.05693970e-04],
          [1.13011487e-01, 2.71215528e-01, 2.30411619e-01, 2.98486114e-01,
          8.68752897e-02],
          [8.86667788e-01, 1.04494877e-01, 6.63056364e-03, 1.91386475e-03,
          2.92797282e-04],
          [8.74389350e-01, 1.14840925e-01, 7.96464831e-03, 2.42676493e-03,
          3.78298369e-04],
          [1.06043883e-01, 2.49819279e-01, 2.38442108e-01, 3.04836661e-01,
          1.00858085e-01],
          [7.40871191e-01, 2.12562516e-01, 3.03196758e-02, 1.36149665e-02,
          2.63170991e-03],
          [7.86449611e-01, 1.81655303e-01, 2.15843264e-02, 8.69893841e-03,
          1.61177712e-03],
          [8.90560150e-01, 1.00513063e-01, 6.71979412e-03, 1.89320825e-03,
          3.13772325e-04],
          [9.03989911e-01, 8.90645757e-02, 5.31880464e-03, 1.40023627e-03,
          2.26360804e-04],
          [8.57582331e-01, 1.28445357e-01, 1.01387231e-02, 3.29650776e-03,
          5.37161250e-04],
          [7.43690312e-01, 2.12609112e-01, 2.85454392e-02, 1.28174732e-02,
          2.33773072e-03],
          [5.92802703e-01, 2.91502774e-01, 6.73934817e-02, 3.95577326e-02,
          8.74337275e-03],
          [1.08115964e-01, 2.47630060e-01, 2.39566654e-01, 3.01667005e-01,
          1.03020266e-01],
          [8.70782733e-01, 1.17978081e-01, 8.27959739e-03, 2.56324536e-03,
          3.96283926e-04],
          [7.59053648e-01, 1.98871464e-01, 2.77820975e-02, 1.19030857e-02,
          2.38960725e-03],
          [8.44498575e-01, 1.34342074e-01, 1.50505928e-02, 4.99778474e-03,
          1.11100485e-03],
          [6.71156108e-01, 2.53151149e-01, 4.66687866e-02, 2.40013525e-02,
          5.02254814e-03],
          [5.33971429e-01, 3.26808959e-01, 7.78735280e-02, 5.12168817e-02,
          1.01292143e-02],
          [8.70443881e-01, 1.17023557e-01, 9.20970365e-03, 2.82991957e-03,
          4.92981286e-04],
          [7.69905508e-01, 1.92171559e-01, 2.52804980e-02, 1.05787218e-02,
          2.06370209e-03],
          [8.30866456e-01, 1.48217812e-01, 1.47424173e-02, 5.21692727e-03,
          9.56410193e-04],
          [9.11621511e-01, 8.25882554e-02, 4.48215613e-03, 1.13246811e-03,
          1.75669353e-04],
          [6.37527823e-01, 2.50932038e-01, 6.66824207e-02, 3.46858911e-02,
          1.01718791e-02],
          [1.02937825e-01, 2.53119171e-01, 2.36675709e-01, 3.09640139e-01,
          9.76271704e-02],
          [1.56325504e-01, 2.95393705e-01, 2.20237121e-01, 2.52701730e-01,
          7.53418878e-02],
          [6.46143198e-01, 2.41424024e-01, 6.74633533e-02, 3.40964533e-02,
          1.08729564e-02],
          [8.39222729e-01, 1.41632959e-01, 1.36041418e-02, 4.68115415e-03,
          8.59017367e-04],
          [1.09037854e-01, 2.46659145e-01, 2.40053445e-01, 3.00265551e-01,
          1.03983983e-01],
          [2.55965441e-01, 3.55194777e-01, 1.74702838e-01, 1.72652677e-01,
          4.14842218e-02],
          [6.73872709e-01, 2.51807630e-01, 4.59172837e-02, 2.35070121e-02,
          4.89531457e-03],
          [9.06672299e-01, 8.71637613e-02, 4.74287709e-03, 1.23610883e-03,
          1.85016863e-04],
          [1.13389641e-01, 2.42101148e-01, 2.42241234e-01, 2.93720275e-01,
          1.08547643e-01],
          [8.09805870e-01, 1.67246982e-01, 1.58957280e-02, 6.08204398e-03,
          9.69371991e-04],
          [7.43020594e-01, 2.11406216e-01, 2.97286324e-02, 1.32969376e-02,
          2.54769134e-03],
          [8.08218479e-01, 1.67094812e-01, 1.70564372e-02, 6.51578791e-03,
          1.11444131e-03],
          [2.43963584e-01, 3.37263972e-01, 1.86235085e-01, 1.83049321e-01,
          4.94880304e-02]], dtype=float32)
```

As we can see in the preceding screenshot, we get the class probabilities for each individual class. We see that there's basically no chance of the higher levels of heart disease. So, we add an `np.argmax` argument, where we mention whichever class has the highest probability and label that as a 1, while everything else will be labeled as 0:

```
In [30]:  # generate classification report using predictions for categorical model
          from sklearn.metrics import classification_report, accuracy_score

          categorical_pred = np.argmax(model.predict(X_test), axis=1)

In [31]:  categorical_pred

Out[31]:  array([3, 0, 0, 3, 3, 3, 0, 1, 0, 3, 0, 3, 0, 0, 0, 0, 1, 3, 0, 0, 0, 0,
                 1, 0, 3, 0, 0, 3, 0, 0, 0, 0, 0, 0, 0, 0, 3, 0, 0, 0, 0, 0, 0, 0,
                 0, 0, 0, 3, 1, 0, 0, 3, 1, 0, 0, 3, 0, 0, 0, 1], dtype=int64)
```

Upon running the code, we see that we actually have all 3s there, which is an issue in terms of accuracy. However, that might just be what we predicted in this particular case. This is probably why we are not doing that well—because we are not actually predicting every single level of coronary artery disease. So, let's actually print out some more detailed results for the categorical model, along with `accuracy_score, y_test, categorical_pred, classification_report, y_test,` and `categorical_pred`:

```
In [39]:  # generate classification report using predictions for categorical model
          from sklearn.metrics import classification_report, accuracy_score

          categorical_pred = np.argmax(model.predict(X_test), axis=1)

          print('Results for Categorical Model')
          print(accuracy_score(y_test, categorical_pred))
          print(classification_report(y_test, categorical_pred))

          Results for Categorical Model
          0.6333333333333333
                        precision    recall  f1-score   support

                     0       0.84      0.86      0.85        36
                     1       0.00      0.00      0.00         9
                     2       0.00      0.00      0.00         5
                     3       0.35      1.00      0.52         7
                     4       0.00      0.00      0.00         3

          avg / total       0.54      0.63      0.57        60
```

So, we can see that we are 66% accurate. There were 11 instances in our testing dataset with level 1 that we should have predicted, but didn't. Similarly, with level 4, there were three cases that we should also have predicted. After this, we had results of 83% and 97% for `precision` and `recall` for our healthy patients. `precision`, of course, tracks false positives. Here, we had a few false positives, where we predicted that a patient was healthy when they weren't. The 97% result for `recall` also showed that we had one false negative for healthy patients. The `f1-score` is a combined `precision` and `recall` score, while `support` is the number of instances that we had. So, we had 60 patients in our testing dataset, of which 39 were healthy. This is not an algorithm that we could use in a healthcare setting.

Now, let's generate a classification report using predictions for the binary model. However, we're going to do this a little bit differently. We will do an `np.round`, which will give us different float values (anywhere between 0 and 1), and we're going to push this round function to 0 if it is under 0.5, and to 1 if it is over 0.5. Then we will print out the results for this, shown as follows:

```
In [40]:    # generate classification report using predictions for binary model
            binary_pred = np.round(binary_model.predict(X_test)).astype(int)

            print('Results for Binary Model')
            print(accuracy_score(Y_test_binary, binary_pred))
            print(classification_report(Y_test_binary, binary_pred))

            Results for Binary Model
            0.8
                           precision    recall  f1-score   support

                        0       0.83      0.83      0.83        36
                        1       0.75      0.75      0.75        24

            avg / total        0.80      0.80      0.80        60
```

As the preceding screenshot demonstrates, we did much better this time, with 78% accuracy overall. This is probably how you'd actually want your algorithm to function in the healthcare field; it would be preferable to play it safe and predict heart disease when there was none, rather than to miss heart disease and tell patients that they are healthy when they are not. Consequently, our combined `f1-scores` are much better than they were in our categorical problem.

Summary

In this chapter, we looked at how to use sklearn and Keras, how to import data from a UCI repository using the pandas `read_csv` function, and how to preprocess that data. One of the ways to handle missing data, whether in healthcare applications or not, is to remove the rows or instances that have missing attributes. We then learned how to describe the data and print out histograms so we know what we're working with, followed by doing a train/test split with `model_selection` from sklearn. Furthermore, we also learned how to convert one-hot encoded vectors for a categorical classification, by defining simple neural networks using Keras. We then looked at types of activation function, such as softmax, for categorical classifications with `categorical_crossentropy`. In contrast, when we got to our binary classification, we used a sigmoid activation function and a `binary_crossentropy` loss. We also looked at training that data and how we fit our model to our training data. We did that for both categorical and binary problems. Then, finally, we looked at how to do a classification report and accuracy score for our results.

In the next chapter, we will learn how to screen children using machine learning to see if they have autism.

Autism Screening with Machine Learning

5

An early diagnosis of neurodevelopmental disorders can improve treatment and significantly decrease associated healthcare costs. In this chapter, we will use supervised learning to diagnose **Autistic Spectrum Disorder** (**ASD**) based on behavioral features and individual characteristics. More specifically, we will build and deploy a neural network using the Keras API.

We will cover the following topics in this chapter:

- ASD screening using machine learning
- Introducing the dataset
- Splitting the dataset into training and testing datasets
- Building the network
- Testing the network
- Solving overfitting issues using dropout regularization

ASD screening using machine learning

We will be using a Jupyter Notebook, which runs on iPython. We will also use the pandas, Keras, and scikit-learn libraries here:

1. To open a Notebook we will use the Command Prompt in Windows.
2. We will first navigate to the directory where our project is present using the cd command, as shown in the following screenshot:

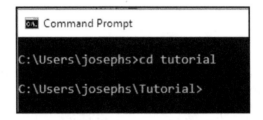

3. Once we are in the required directory, we will open up Jupyter Lab using the following command:

```
jupyter lab
```

4. When we press *Enter* after this command, we will see the Notebook open. Here, we will see that there's an untitled file open in the Notebook. We will then rename that file to autism_detection.

Ctrl + B will close the directory window present on the left side. This will expand your Notebook so that it takes up the whole screen.

Introducing the dataset

The dataset that we're going to be using for this chapter is the Autistic Spectrum Disorder Screening Data for Children Dataset provided by the UCI Machine Learning Repository, which can be found here: https://archive.ics.uci.edu/ml/datasets/ Autistic+Spectrum+Disorder+Screening+Data+for+Children++. This dataset contains records of 292 patients or children that have been screened for autism. This contains details of their age, ethnicity, and familial history of autism. We will be using this dataset to predict whether these patients actually have autism.

Now, we have to download the ZIP file present in the repository and extract the contents. In this zip file, we will find two files. The first file contains a description of the attributes present in the dataset. This file mentions the different features that we'll be using for predictions in this chapter. It tells us a little bit about how the data was collected, and gives us some source information. We will find some information about the tasks that this can be used for and its attribute types. We may find that the dataset contains missing values; this issue will be addressed later in this chapter. The file also gives some information about the actual attributes, as mentioned in the following table:

Attribute	Type	Description
Age	Number	years
Gender	String	Male or Female
Ethnicity	String	List of common ethnicities in text format
Born with jaundice	Boolean (yes or no)	Whether the case was born with jaundice
Family member with PDD	Boolean (yes or no)	Whether any immediate family member has a PDD
Who is completing the test	String	Parent, self, caregiver, medical staff, clinician, etc.
Country of residence	String	List of countries in text format
Used the screening app before	Boolean (yes or no)	Whether the user has used a screening app
Screening Method Type	Integer (0,1,2,3)	The type of screening methods chosen based on age category (0=toddler, 1=child, 2= adolescent, 3= adult)
Question 1 Answer	Binary (0, 1)	The answer code of the question based on the screening method used
Question 2 Answer	Binary (0, 1)	The answer code of the question based on the screening method used
Question 3 Answer	Binary (0, 1)	The answer code of the question based on the screening method used
Question 4 Answer	Binary (0, 1)	The answer code of the question based on the screening method used
Question 5 Answer	Binary (0, 1)	The answer code of the question based on the screening method used
Question 6 Answer	Binary (0, 1)	The answer code of the question based on the screening method used
Question 7 Answer	Binary (0, 1)	The answer code of the question based on the screening method used
Question 8 Answer	Binary (0, 1)	The answer code of the question based on the screening method used
Question 9 Answer	Binary (0, 1)	The answer code of the question based on the screening method used
Question 10 Answer	Binary (0, 1)	The answer code of the question based on the screening method used
Screening Score	Integer	The final score obtained based on the scoring algorithm of the screening method used. This was computed in an automated manner

Here, we can see different attributes such as age, gender, ethnicity, and whether or not the child was born with jaundice. There are also certain questions that have a positive or negative answer (0 or 1). Typically, a psychologist would look at these answers and then meet the child, talk to them about their family history, take other risk factors into account, and then make a decision as to whether that child has autism.

We will now try automating this process using a machine learning algorithm, or more specifically, a neural network.

We also have the ARFF file, and we will open this as a Notepad file. From here, we will see that this file just contains text. So in this file, we see the attributes that we were discussing earlier and, when we scroll down, we will find the data that will be used in this chapter.

We will now save this file in the directory where our project is. After saving, we have to edit this ARFF file a little bit.

When we're importing this, we have to specify that the information is delineated or separated by commas. That shouldn't be hard to do. We have to get rid of all the content that is software-specific in these ARFF files, including the present `@attribute` lines. The data then starts at the first line. We'll then save it as a text file and simply import this file straight into the Jupyter Notebook.

Importing the data and libraries

Now, let's return to our Jupyter Notebook.

We will now import the dataset and the libraries into our Jupyter Notebook using the following steps:

1. If we go into **Files**, we will see all the files that we have in the directory, as shown in the following screenshot:

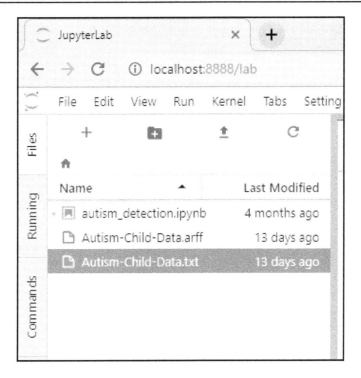

Here, we have the ARFF file and the text version that we just saved, as well as our Jupyter Notebook. Let's get started with this.

2. We will now import the following libraries and print their version numbers:

```
import sys
import pandas as pd
import sklearn
import keras
print 'Python: {}'.format(sys.version)
print 'Pandas: {}'.format(pd.__version__)
print 'Sklearn: {}'.format(sklearn.__version__)
print 'Keras: {}'.format(keras.__version__)
```

This will generate output that is similar to the following screenshot:

```
In [1]:  import sys
         import pandas as pd
         import sklearn
         import keras

         print 'Python: {}'.format(sys.version)
         print 'Pandas: {}'.format(pd.__version__)
         print 'Sklearn: {}'.format(sklearn.__version__)
         print 'Keras: {}'.format(keras.__version__)

         Using Theano backend.
         WARNING (theano.tensor.blas): Using NumPy C-API based implementation for BLAS functions.

         Python: 2.7.13 |Continuum Analytics, Inc.| (default, May 11 2017, 13:17:26) [MSC v.1500 64 bit (AMD64)]
         Pandas: 0.21.0
         Sklearn: 0.19.1
         Keras: 2.1.4
```

3. Now, let's import the autism dataset. To do that, we will define the `Autism-Child-Data.txt` file that we saved earlier.

4. Then, we will read this into the Notebook using `pandas`.

The following lines of code show how it is done:

```
# import the dataset
file = 'C:/users/brend/tutorial/autism-data.txt'
# read the csv
data = pd.read_table(file, sep = ',', index_col = None)
```

Exploring the dataset

Now, let's actually explore the dataset so that we can see what information we have. In order to do that, we're going to print the shape of the DataFrame so that we can see how many examples are present in the dataset. We will use the following lines of code to do that:

```
# print the shape of the DataFrame, so we can see how many examples we have
print 'Shape of DataFrame: {}'.format(data.shape)
print data.loc[0]
```

This will generate the following output:

```
Shape of DataFrame: (292, 21)
A1_Score                                    1
A2_Score                                    1
A3_Score                                    0
A4_Score                                    0
A5_Score                                    1
A6_Score                                    1
A7_Score                                    0
A8_Score                                    1
A9_Score                                    0
A10_Score                                   0
age_numeric                                 6
gender                                      m
ethnicity                              Others
jaundice                                   no
family_history_of_autism                   no
country_of_res                         Jordan
used_app_before                            no
result                                      5
age_desc                          '4-11 years'
relation                               Parent
Class/ASD                                  NO
Name: 0, dtype: object
```

We have 292 patients with 21 attributes each, one of those being the Class label. So, we have our 10 scores, which we saw in our text file, namely age, gender, ethnicity, jaundice, and family_history_of_autism. Furthermore, we find that a particular patient [0] who does not have autism is a six-year-old child who lives in Jordan.

Let's print out records for the first eleven patients. To do that, we can use the `data.loc[]` method, as shown in the following screenshot:

	A1_Score	A2_Score	A3_Score	A4_Score	A5_Score	A6_Score	A7_Score	A8_Score	A9_Score	A10_Score	...	gender	ethnicity	jaundice	family_history_of_autism	country_of_res	used_app_before
0	1	1	0	0	1	1	0	1	0	0	...	m	Others	no	no	Jordan	no
1	1	1	0	0	1	1	0	1	0	0	...	m	'Middle Eastern '	no	no	Jordan	no
2	1	1	0	0	0	1	1	1	0	0	...	m	?	no	no	Jordan	yes
3	0	1	0	0	1	1	0	0	0	1	...	f	?	yes	no	Jordan	no
4	1	1	1	1	1	1	1	1	1	1	...	m	Others	yes	no	United States'	no
5	0	0	1	0	1	1	0	1	0	1	...	m	?	no	yes	Egypt	no
6	1	0	1	1	1	1	0	1	0	1	...	m	White-European	no	no	'United Kingdom'	no
7	1	1	1	1	1	1	1	1	0	0	...	f	'Middle Eastern '	no	no	Bahrain	no
8	1	1	1	1	1	1	1	0	0	0	...	f	'Middle Eastern '	no	no	Bahrain	no
9	0	0	1	1	1	0	1	1	0	0	...	f	?	no	yes	Austria	no
10	1	0	0	0	1	1	1	1	1	1	...	m	White-European	yes	no	'United Kingdom'	no

11 rows × 21 columns

The first eleven patients and their data are listed in the preceding screenshot. However, we do notice that some patients have not provided data regarding their ethnicity. Those data fields have question marks.

Now, let's print out a DataFrame that gives us a lot of helpful information for the dataset. This is done with the help of the `describe()` function, which gives you information such as the mean, min, max, and so on for all numerical data. This can be seen in the following screenshot:

```
In [17]: # print out a description of the dataframe
         data.describe()
```

	A1_Score	A2_Score	A3_Score	A4_Score	A5_Score	A6_Score	A7_Score	A8_Score	A9_Score	A10_Score	result
count	292.000000	292.000000	292.000000	292.000000	292.000000	292.000000	292.000000	292.000000	292.000000	292.000000	292.000000
mean	0.633562	0.534247	0.743151	0.551370	0.743151	0.712329	0.606164	0.496575	0.493151	0.726027	6.239726
std	0.482658	0.499682	0.437646	0.498208	0.437646	0.453454	0.489438	0.500847	0.500811	0.446761	2.284882
min	0.000000	0.000000	0.000000	0.000000	0.000000	0.000000	0.000000	0.000000	0.000000	0.000000	0.000000
25%	0.000000	0.000000	0.000000	0.000000	0.000000	0.000000	0.000000	0.000000	0.000000	0.000000	5.000000
50%	1.000000	1.000000	1.000000	1.000000	1.000000	1.000000	1.000000	0.000000	0.000000	1.000000	6.000000
75%	1.000000	1.000000	1.000000	1.000000	1.000000	1.000000	1.000000	1.000000	1.000000	1.000000	8.000000
max	1.000000	1.000000	1.000000	1.000000	1.000000	1.000000	1.000000	1.000000	1.000000	1.000000	10.000000

Something that could be helpful here is the ability to see which columns contain numerical data, and this `describe()` function will showcase that. An alternative way of finding information about the data types is by using the following line:

```
data.dtypes
```

This gives us the following result:

```
In [24]: data.dtypes

Out[24]: A1_Score                      int64
         A2_Score                      int64
         A3_Score                      int64
         A4_Score                      int64
         A5_Score                      int64
         A6_Score                      int64
         A7_Score                      int64
         A8_Score                      int64
         A9_Score                      int64
         A10_Score                     int64
         age_numeric                  object
         gender                       object
         ethnicity                    object
         jaundice                     object
         family_history_of_autism     object
         country_of_res               object
         used_app_before              object
         result                        int64
         age_desc                     object
         relation                     object
         Class/ASD                    object
         dtype: object
```

In the preceding screenshot, we can see that the columns from `A1_Score` to `A10_Score` are integers. However, all others are objects. The `age numeric` column is an object because we have some missing data in our `age numeric` column, which we will be correcting soon. The `gender` and `ethnicity` columns are all objects because these are all strings and question marks.

> An object is pandas' way of saying that there are multiple data types in a particular column.

Data preprocessing

Now, we'll look at preprocessing and what we have to do to handle that. We actually don't need all of the information present in the dataset. The age description is not needed because all of these individuals are between 4 and 11 years, and this is the same for all patients. So we will now drop the `age_desc` column using the following steps:

1. We're going to go ahead and drop the `age_desc` column. Also, let's go ahead and drop the `result numeric` column since it is a weighted calculation of the screening method based on responses to the questions mentioned earlier. We have to make sure that we're not predicting whether these children have autism based on this column alone. To actually drop the columns, we will use the following lines of code:

   ```
   # drop unwanted columns
   data = data.drop(['result numeric', 'age_desc'], axis=1)
   ```

2. When we run the `loc()` function again, we can see that the `result numeric` and `age_desc` columns have been removed from the DataFrame.

3. Our next step is to split the DataFrame into two datasets, x and y . Here, x is going to represent all of the attributes that we'll use for prediction and y is going to be our `Class/ASD` label.

   We will split the DataFrame by using the following lines of code:

   ```
   x = data.drop(['Class/ASD'], 1)
   y = data['Class/ASD']
   ```

4. Now, we will print out the x dataset to see the changes we have made. This is done by using the `loc[]` function, as shown in the following screenshot:

	A1_Score	A2_Score	A3_Score	A4_Score	A5_Score	A6_Score	A7_Score	A8_Score	A9_Score	A10_Score	age_numeric	gender	ethnicity	jaundice	family_history_of_autism	country_of_res	used_app_be
0	1	1	0	0	1	1	0	1	0	0	6	m	Others	no	no	Jordan	
1	1	1	0	0	1	1	0	1	0	0	6	m	'Middle Eastern '	no	no	Jordan	
2	1	1	0	0	0	1	1	1	0	0	6	m	?	no	no	Jordan	
3	0	1	0	0	1	1	0	0	0	1	5	f	?	yes	no	Jordan	
4	1	1	1	1	1	1	1	1	1	1	5	m	Others	yes	no	'United States'	
5	0	0	1	0	1	1	0	1	0	1	4	m	?	no	yes	Egypt	
6	1	0	1	1	1	1	0	1	0	1	5	m	White-European	no	no	'United Kingdom'	
7	1	1	1	1	1	1	1	1	0	0	5	f	'Middle Eastern'	no	no	Bahrain	
8	1	1	1	1	1	1	1	0	0	0	11	f	'Middle Eastern'	no	no	Bahrain	
9	0	0	1	1	1	0	1	1	0	0	11	f	?	no	yes	Austria	
10	1	0	0	0	1	1	1	1	1	1	10	m	White-European	yes	no	'United Kingdom'	

In the preceding screenshot, we can see that there's no `Class/ASD` column in the dataset.

One-hot encoding

Now, we need to take care of the fact that we have values such as `Others`, `Middle Eastern`, and a `?` all in the same column. We will have to convert the data to categorical variables so that the machine learning algorithm can read them. These variables are also called **one-hot encoded vectors** and they can be created easily using `pandas`:

1. All we need to do is use the `get_dummies` function. This will convert the values in the x dataset to categorical variables and show the dummy values. This is done using the following line:

```
X = pd.get_dummies(x)
```

2. Now, if we print out the DataFrame, we won't be able to see everything in the window because there are many more columns present. Instead, we will print out the values for all the columns to see what we are getting. This is shown in the following screenshot:

```
In [54]:  # print the new categorical column labels
          X.columns.values

Out[54]:  array(['A1_Score', ' A2_Score', ' A3_Score', ' A4_Score', ' A5_Score',
                 ' A6_Score', ' A7_Score', ' A8_Score', ' A9_Score', ' A10_Score',
                 ' age_numeric_10', ' age_numeric_11', ' age_numeric_4',
                 ' age_numeric_5', ' age_numeric_6', ' age_numeric_7',
                 ' age_numeric_8', ' age_numeric_9', ' age_numeric_?', ' gender_f',
                 ' gender_m', " ethnicity_'Middle Eastern '",
                 " ethnicity_'South Asian'", ' ethnicity_?', ' ethnicity_Asian',
                 ' ethnicity_Black', ' ethnicity_Hispanic', ' ethnicity_Latino',
                 ' ethnicity_Others', ' ethnicity_Pasifika', ' ethnicity_Turkish',
                 ' ethnicity_White-European', ' jaundice_no', ' jaundice_yes',
                 ' family_history_of_autism_no', ' family_history_of_autism_yes',
                 " country_of_res_'Costa Rica'", " country_of_res_'Isle of Man'",
                 " country_of_res_'New Zealand'", " country_of_res_'Saudi Arabia'",
                 " country_of_res_'South Africa'", " country_of_res_'South Korea'",
                 " country_of_res_'U.S. Outlying Islands'",
                 " country_of_res_'United Arab Emirates'",
                 " country_of_res_'United Kingdom'",
                 " country_of_res_'United States'", ' country_of_res_Afghanistan',
                 ' country_of_res_Argentina', ' country_of_res_Armenia',
                 ' country_of_res_Australia', ' country_of_res_Austria',
                 ' country_of_res_Bahrain', ' country_of_res_Bangladesh',
                 ' country_of_res_Bhutan', ' country_of_res_Brazil',
                 ' country_of_res_Bulgaria', ' country_of_res_Canada',
                 ' country_of_res_China', ' country_of_res_Egypt',
                 ' country_of_res_Europe', ' country_of_res_Georgia',
                 ' country_of_res_Germany', ' country_of_res_Ghana',
                 ' country_of_res_India', ' country_of_res_Iraq',
                 ' country_of_res_Ireland', ' country_of_res_Italy',
                 ' country_of_res_Japan', ' country_of_res_Jordan',
                 ' country_of_res_Kuwait', ' country_of_res_Latvia',
                 ' country_of_res_Lebanon', ' country_of_res_Libya',
                 ' country_of_res_Malaysia', ' country_of_res_Malta',
                 ' country_of_res_Mexico', ' country_of_res_Nepal',
                 ' country_of_res_Netherlands', ' country_of_res_Nigeria',
                 ' country_of_res_Oman', ' country_of_res_Pakistan',
                 ' country_of_res_Philippines', ' country_of_res_Qatar',
                 ' country_of_res_Romania', ' country_of_res_Russia',
                 ' country_of_res_Sweden', ' country_of_res_Syria',
                 ' country_of_res_Turkey', ' used_app_before_no',
                 ' used_app_before_yes', " relation_'Health care professional'",
                 ' relation_?', ' relation_Parent', ' relation_Relative',
                 ' relation_Self', ' relation_self'], dtype=object)
```

We see that there are a large number of columns present for each data element. Let's consider the example of the `age numeric` column. When the patient doesn't fill out his/her age, then there will be a `1` in the `age numeric_?` column. If the patient does fill out their age, then the column pertaining to that age will have a value of `1` in it.

3. Now, let's print out an example for one patient. To do that, we will again use the `loc[]` function. This operation is shown in the following screenshot:

```
In [19]:  # print an example patient from the categorical data
          X.loc[1]
```

```
Out[19]:  A1_Score                          1     contry_of_res_ Italy                            0
          A2_Score                          1     contry_of_res_ Japan                            0
          A3_Score                          0     contry_of_res_ Jordan                           1
          A4_Score                          0     contry_of_res_ Kuwait                           0
          A5_Score                          1     contry_of_res_ Latvia                           0
          A6_Score                          1     contry_of_res_ Lebanon                          0
          A7_Score                          0     contry_of_res_ Libya                            0
          A8_Score                          1     contry_of_res_ Malaysia                         0
          A9_Score                          0     contry_of_res_ Malta                            0
          A10_Score                         0     contry_of_res_ Mexico                           0
          age numeric_ 10                   0     contry_of_res_ Nepal                            0
          age numeric_ 11                   0     contry_of_res_ Netherlands                      0
          age numeric_ 4                    0     contry_of_res_ Nigeria                          0
          age numeric_ 5                    0     contry_of_res_ Oman                             0
          age numeric_ 6                    1     contry_of_res_ Pakistan                         0
          age numeric_ 7                    0     contry_of_res_ Philippines                      0
          age numeric_ 8                    0     contry_of_res_ Qatar                            0
          age numeric_ 9                    0     contry_of_res_ Romania                          0
          age numeric_ ?                    0     contry_of_res_ Russia                           0
          gender_ f                         0     contry_of_res_ Sweden                           0
          gender_ m                         1     contry_of_res_ Syria                            0
          ethnicity_ 'Middle Eastern '      1     contry_of_res_ Turkey                           0
          ethnicity_ 'South Asian'          0     used_app_before_ no                             1
          ethnicity_ ?                      0     used_app_before_ yes                            0
          ethnicity_ Asian                  0     relation_ 'Health care professional'            0
          ethnicity_ Black                  0     relation_ ?                                     0
          ethnicity_ Hispanic               0     relation_ Parent                                1
          ethnicity_ Latino                 0     relation_ Relative                              0
          ethnicity_ Others                 0     relation_ Self                                  0
          ethnicity_ Pasifika               0     relation_ self                                  0
                                          ..      Name: 1, Length: 96, dtype: int64
```

4. We have to do the same thing for our y dataset. This process follows the same steps that we followed for the x dataset. The output is shown in the following screenshot:

```
In [20]:  # convert the class data to categorical values - one-hot-encoded vectors
          Y = pd.get_dummies(y)

In [21]:  Y.iloc[:10]

Out[21]:
                NO   YES
          0      1    0
          1      1    0
          2      1    0
          3      1    0
          4      0    1
          5      1    0
          6      0    1
          7      0    1
          8      0    1
          9      1    0
```

The output in the preceding screenshot is going to be fed directly into our neural network during our training phase. This entire process is called the **one-hot encoding** process.

Splitting the dataset into training and testing datasets

Before we can begin training our neural network, we need to split the dataset into training and testing datasets. This will allow us to test our network after we are done training in order to determine how well it will generalize new data. This step is incredibly easy when using the `train_test_split()` function provided by `scikit-learn`. So, we reserve some of the data that we have to test so that we can see how well our algorithm is performing.

1. To do that, we will import the `model_selection` package from `sklearn`. From this package, we're going to use the `train_test_split` function. The following lines of code show us how to split the data into the required training and testing sets:

```
from sklearn import model_selection
# split the X and Y data into training and testing datasets
X_train, X_test, Y_train, Y_test =
model_selection.train_test_split(X, Y, test_size = 0.2)
```

We will assume that the testing dataset contains 20% of the data that will be used for training the network.

2. Consequently, we take the `test_size` value as `0.2`. After we split the datasets, we will now print the shape of the datasets to see how many attributes are split between them. This is shown in the following screenshot:

```
In [24]:  print(X_train.shape)
          print (X_test.shape)
          print (Y_train.shape)
          print (Y_test.shape)

          (233, 96)
          (59, 96)
          (233, 2)
          (59, 2)
```

As seen with the x dataset, `233` of our patients are in the training dataset and `59` are in the testing dataset, each of which has `96` attributes. As for our y dataset, we only have `2` attributes here because we have two options for the class labels.

Building the network

We are now done with the data preprocessing that is necessary to prepare the data for machine learning. Now, it's time to start the fun part, where we actually get to build a neural network. We will train it using our training data, and then test it on our testing dataset:

1. Let's go ahead and import the layers and models that we need to build the model. The following lines of code show all the imported layers:

```
from keras.models import Sequential
from keras.layers import Dense
from keras.optimizers import Adam
```

In the preceding code snippet, Adam is the standard optimizer that people use with deep neural networks and Keras.

2. The next step is defining a function to build the Keras model, which can be done via the create_model() function. This function also gives us a way to replicate the model with slightly different parameters by defining inputs.

3. Now, we have to create the model using the following lines of code:

```
def create_model():
 # create model
 model = Sequential()
 model.add(Dense(8, input_dim=96, kernel_initializer='normal',
activation='relu'))
 model.add(Dense(4, kernel_initializer='normal',
activation='relu'))
 model.add(Dense(2, activation='sigmoid'))
```

4. Our next step will be compiling the model. To do that, we first need to define an optimizer and specify a learning rate for it. Here, we will use the Adam optimizer with a learning rate of 0.001. Then, we have to compile the model by specifying a loss function, an optimizer, and the performance metrics that we will be using. Furthermore, we have to use the return command since the entire code block is just a function. The following code block shows us how we will compile and return the model:

```
 # compile model
 adam = Adam(lr=0.001)
 model.compile(loss='categorical_crossentropy', optimizer=adam,
metrics=['accuracy'])
 return model
```

In the preceding code snippet, the loss function will be the
`categorical_crossentropy` loss function. We also defined the Adam
optimizer and assigned accuracy performance metrics to the model.

5. Now that we have defined the model, we have to create it by calling the
`create_model` function that we defined in the previous steps. After this, we will
print out the model using the `print()` function, as seen in the following
screenshot:

```
In [34]:  model = create_model()
          print(model.summary())

          _____
          Layer (type)                 Output Shape              Param #
          =================================================================
          dense_4 (Dense)              (None, 8)                 776
          _____
          dense_5 (Dense)              (None, 4)                 36
          _____
          dense_6 (Dense)              (None, 2)                 10
          =================================================================
          Total params: 822
          Trainable params: 822
          Non-trainable params: 0
          _____
          None
```

As we can see, we have created a neural network consisting of three layers, where
the first layer has 8 neurons, the second layer has 4 neurons, and the third layer
has 2 neurons. From this, we can see that there are 822 trainable parameters in
the network.

6. Now that we have the network, here's the cool step. We need to fit the model to
the training data. To do that in Keras, we have to use the `model.fit()` function.
This is supervised learning, which means that we will provide labels during the
training phase. We will define the `epochs` as 50 since we want the model to go
through the data 50 times. From this point, we will define the `batch_size` as 10
since we want the model to work with the first 10 patients only. The following
line of code shows the complete `fit()` function along with all the parameters:

```
model.fit(X_train, Y_train, epochs=50, batch_size=10, verbose = 1)
```

An entire round or pass through each of the training instances (patients) is referred to as an epoch.

This results in the following output:

```
Epoch 1/50                                                              Epoch 26/50
233/233 [==============================] - 0s 288us/step - loss: 0.6927 - acc: 0.5794   233/233 [==============================] - 0s 339us/step - loss: 0.0585 - acc: 0.9957
Epoch 2/50                                                              Epoch 27/50
233/233 [==============================] - 0s 245us/step - loss: 0.6910 - acc: 0.7210   233/233 [==============================] - 0s 335us/step - loss: 0.0571 - acc: 1.0000
Epoch 3/50                                                              Epoch 28/50
233/233 [==============================] - 0s 258us/step - loss: 0.6868 - acc: 0.7639   233/233 [==============================] - 0s 429us/step - loss: 0.0526 - acc: 0.9957
Epoch 4/50                                                              Epoch 29/50
233/233 [==============================] - 0s 236us/step - loss: 0.6779 - acc: 0.7082   233/233 [==============================] - 0s 335us/step - loss: 0.0474 - acc: 1.0000
Epoch 5/50                                                              Epoch 30/50
233/233 [==============================] - 0s 236us/step - loss: 0.6619 - acc: 0.8541   233/233 [==============================] - 0s 322us/step - loss: 0.0463 - acc: 0.9957
Epoch 6/50                                                              Epoch 31/50
233/233 [==============================] - 0s 305us/step - loss: 0.6340 - acc: 0.8283   233/233 [==============================] - 0s 296us/step - loss: 0.0431 - acc: 1.0000
Epoch 7/50                                                              Epoch 32/50
233/233 [==============================] - 0s 227us/step - loss: 0.5963 - acc: 0.8541   233/233 [==============================] - 0s 348us/step - loss: 0.0381 - acc: 1.0000
Epoch 8/50                                                              Epoch 33/50
233/233 [==============================] - 0s 305us/step - loss: 0.5446 - acc: 0.9399   233/233 [==============================] - 0s 322us/step - loss: 0.0357 - acc: 1.0000
Epoch 9/50                                                              Epoch 34/50
233/233 [==============================] - 0s 240us/step - loss: 0.4884 - acc: 0.8884   233/233 [==============================] - 0s 292us/step - loss: 0.0331 - acc: 1.0000
Epoch 10/50                                                             Epoch 35/50
233/233 [==============================] - 0s 227us/step - loss: 0.4220 - acc: 0.9227   233/233 [==============================] - 0s 305us/step - loss: 0.0316 - acc: 1.0000
Epoch 11/50                                                             Epoch 36/50
233/233 [==============================] - 0s 322us/step - loss: 0.3603 - acc: 0.9313   233/233 [==============================] - 0s 335us/step - loss: 0.0294 - acc: 1.0000
Epoch 12/50                                                             Epoch 37/50
233/233 [==============================] - 0s 245us/step - loss: 0.2935 - acc: 0.9614   233/233 [==============================] - 0s 322us/step - loss: 0.0282 - acc: 1.0000
Epoch 13/50                                                             Epoch 38/50
233/233 [==============================] - 0s 296us/step - loss: 0.2528 - acc: 0.9657   233/233 [==============================] - 0s 236us/step - loss: 0.0281 - acc: 1.0000
Epoch 14/50                                                             Epoch 39/50
233/233 [==============================] - 0s 330us/step - loss: 0.2087 - acc: 0.9657   233/233 [==============================] - 0s 339us/step - loss: 0.0253 - acc: 1.0000
Epoch 15/50                                                             Epoch 40/50
233/233 [==============================] - 0s 305us/step - loss: 0.1788 - acc: 0.9871   233/233 [==============================] - 0s 223us/step - loss: 0.0252 - acc: 1.0000
Epoch 16/50                                                             Epoch 41/50
233/233 [==============================] - 0s 313us/step - loss: 0.1605 - acc: 0.9700   233/233 [==============================] - 0s 326us/step - loss: 0.0226 - acc: 1.0000
Epoch 17/50                                                             Epoch 42/50
233/233 [==============================] - 0s 309us/step - loss: 0.1389 - acc: 0.9828   233/233 [==============================] - 0s 326us/step - loss: 0.0213 - acc: 1.0000
Epoch 18/50                                                             Epoch 43/50
233/233 [==============================] - 0s 335us/step - loss: 0.1258 - acc: 0.9785   233/233 [==============================] - 0s 219us/step - loss: 0.0203 - acc: 1.0000
Epoch 19/50                                                             Epoch 44/50
233/233 [==============================] - 0s 343us/step - loss: 0.1108 - acc: 0.9871   233/233 [==============================] - 0s 215us/step - loss: 0.0193 - acc: 1.0000
Epoch 20/50                                                             Epoch 45/50
233/233 [==============================] - 0s 399us/step - loss: 0.1004 - acc: 0.9871   233/233 [==============================] - 0s 318us/step - loss: 0.0190 - acc: 1.0000
Epoch 21/50                                                             Epoch 46/50
233/233 [==============================] - 0s 416us/step - loss: 0.0910 - acc: 0.9871   233/233 [==============================] - 0s 232us/step - loss: 0.0176 - acc: 1.0000
Epoch 22/50                                                             Epoch 47/50
233/233 [==============================] - 0s 343us/step - loss: 0.0820 - acc: 0.9871   233/233 [==============================] - 0s 215us/step - loss: 0.0163 - acc: 1.0000
Epoch 23/50                                                             Epoch 48/50
233/233 [==============================] - 0s 361us/step - loss: 0.0752 - acc: 0.9914   233/233 [==============================] - 0s 202us/step - loss: 0.0161 - acc: 1.0000
Epoch 24/50                                                             Epoch 49/50
233/233 [==============================] - 0s 356us/step - loss: 0.0714 - acc: 0.9957   233/233 [==============================] - 0s 240us/step - loss: 0.0154 - acc: 1.0000
Epoch 25/50                                                             Epoch 50/50
233/233 [==============================] - 0s 309us/step - loss: 0.0634 - acc: 0.9957   233/233 [==============================] - 0s 223us/step - loss: 0.0150 - acc: 1.0000
```

In the preceding screenshot, we can see that we started with a pretty low accuracy, but as our accuracy goes up, our loss goes down. Consequently, we find that our accuracy becomes 100% within the first 50 epochs. However, this refers to the accuracy of the training data only.

Testing the network

What we need to see is whether or not this model can now generalize new information, which is why we reserved the testing dataset earlier. We need to generate a classification report using predictions from the model. To do this, we're going to import the `classification_report` and the `accuracy_score` features from the `sklearn.metrics` library. We also have to predict the values, which is very easy to do using the `model.predict()` function. We have to print those out and see what we have. The following lines of code show the process of testing the predictions:

```
# generate classification report using predictions for categorical model
from sklearn.metrics import classification_report, accuracy_score
predictions = model.predict_classes(X_test)
predictions
```

The preceding code snippet generates an array consisting of 1s and 0s, as shown in the following screenshot:

```
In [25]:  # generate classification report using predictions for categorical model
          from sklearn.metrics import classification_report, accuracy_score

          predictions = model.predict_classes(X_test)
          predictions
Out[25]:  array([0, 0, 1, 1, 1, 0, 1, 1, 0, 0, 0, 0, 0, 1, 0, 0, 0, 0, 1, 1, 1, 1,
                 0, 0, 1, 0, 0, 0, 0, 0, 1, 0, 1, 0, 0, 1, 0, 0, 1, 1, 1, 1, 1, 1,
                 0, 1, 1, 0, 1, 0, 0, 0, 1, 0, 1, 1, 1, 0, 0], dtype=int64)
```

Now, let's print out some of our results. We will use the following lines of code to do that:

```
print('Prediction Results for Neural Network')
print(accuracy_score(Y_test[['YES']], predictions))
print(classification_report(Y_test[['YES']], predictions))
```

The following screenshot shows us this result:

```
Prediction Results for Neural Network
0.8983050847457628
               precision    recall  f1-score   support

           0       0.85      0.97      0.90        29
           1       0.96      0.83      0.89        30

avg / total        0.91      0.90      0.90        59
```

With reference to the preceding screenshot, we can see that we are at 90% accuracy right off the bat. We find that `precision` is going to be a false positive while `recall` takes into account false negatives. The `f1-score` is a combined score of those precision and recall scores. The `support` value shows the total number of patients that did or didn't have autism in our testing dataset. We had 30 patients that had autism and 29 who didn't. This shows that the precision of our autism class is accurate, which means that, if a patient does have autism, we're likely to predict it. Similarly, we had very few false positives, which also means that we're very likely to predict when somebody doesn't have autism. We do have some false negatives though, so we missed a few particular examples.

One thing we notice is that we had 100% accuracy on our training dataset, but as soon as we moved to the testing dataset we had 90% accuracy, which is a pretty big drop-off. This essentially means that we're overfitting our network to the training data.

 Overfitting is just a way of saying that we learned the training data so well, and we adjusted our parameters so significantly, that we can no longer generalize new information.

Solving overfitting issues using dropout regularization

This is just a bonus step that you can perform to reduce overfitting. One way to reduce overfitting is via dropout regularization:

1. To do that, let's import `Dropout` from the `keras.layers` library. This `Dropout` function periodically knocks out some of the neurons in the layer to make the other neurons pick up the slack. This is called a **regularization** technique because it's a way to regularize outputs that the neurons are making, and it'll help our network generalize slightly better.

2. We'll define the dropout rate as `0.25` as we have only four neurons before testing starts. This will give us an even value that we can knock out each time. This is done by adding the following line to the model building code block that we created earlier:

```
model.add(Dropout(0.25))
```

Once the dropout layer is created, we will retrain and test the model. Unfortunately, in our case, we don't see much improvement in our accuracy. Dropout works only in certain cases when our data isn't too complicated.

Summary

In this chapter, we were able to predict autism in patients with about 90% accuracy. We also learned how to deal with categorical data; a lot of health applications are going to have categorical data and one way to address this is by using one-hot encoded vectors. Furthermore, we learned how to reduce overfitting using dropout regularization.

In this book, we explored how to implement machine learning to analyze various healthcare issues. In the first chapter, we used machine learning to detect cancer in a set of patients using the SVM and KNN models. In the second chapter, we created a deep neural network in Keras to predict the onset of diabetes on a huge dataset of patients. In the third chapter, we predicted whether or not a short sequence of E.coli bacteria DNA was a promoter or a non-promoter, and we used some common classifiers to classify short E. coli DNA sequences. In the fourth chapter, we predicted heart disease using neural networks. Consequently, we can now see how machine learning in this day and age is revolutionizing the process of detecting the numerous diseases that are prevalent in the field of healthcare.

Another Book You May Enjoy

If you enjoyed this book, you may be interested in another book by Packt:

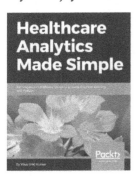

Healthcare Analytics Made Simple
Vikas "Vik" Kumar

ISBN: 978-1-78728-670-2

- Gain valuable insight into healthcare incentives, finances, and legislation
- Discover the connection between machine learning and healthcare processes
- Use SQL and Python to analyze data
- Measure healthcare quality and provider performance
- Identify features and attributes to build successful healthcare models
- Build predictive models using real-world healthcare data
- Become an expert in predictive modeling with structured clinical data
- See what lies ahead for healthcare analytics

Leave a review - let other readers know what you think

Please share your thoughts on this book with others by leaving a review on the site that you bought it from. If you purchased the book from Amazon, please leave us an honest review on this book's Amazon page. This is vital so that other potential readers can see and use your unbiased opinion to make purchasing decisions, we can understand what our customers think about our products, and our authors can see your feedback on the title that they have worked with Packt to create. It will only take a few minutes of your time, but is valuable to other potential customers, our authors, and Packt. Thank you!

Index

training 90, 93
neurons
  number of neurons, optimizing 56, 58

O

one-hot encoded vectors 111
optimal hyperparameters
  searching 53, 55, 56
  used, for generating predictions 58, 60
overfitting
  reducing, with dropout regularization 47, 49, 52

P

predictions
  example 60
  generating, with optimal hyperparameters 58, 60

R

regularization 121

S

scikit-learn
  used, for performing grid search 42, 45, 47
series 65
support vector classifier (SVC) 13
support vector machine (SVM)
  about 9, 11, 15, 18
  used, for detecting breast cancer 9, 11, 15, 18

T

training models 22, 24

www.ingramcontent.com/pod-product-compliance
Lightning Source LLC
Chambersburg PA
CBHW080537060326
40690CB00022B/5157